EVOLUTION HEALTH

How to get healthier by honoring your past and protecting our future!

Edward F. Cotter Jr.

Two Great writer's advice on how to write:

"I wrote you this long letter because I did not have the time to write you a short one." Attributed to Mark Twain.

""I would stand ... and think, "Do not worry. You have always written before and you will write now. All you have to do is write one true sentence. Write the truest sentence that you know." So finally I would write one true sentence and go on from there." "" Ernest Hemingway, *A Movable Feast* at page 12 (1964)

"I had learned already never to empty the well of my writing, but always to stop when there was still something there in the deep part of the well, and let it refill at night from the springs that fed it." *A Movable Feast* at page 26 (1964)

Summary-

Keep it short, keep it honest and keep yourself fresh.

CONTENTS

Part One- My personal journey back to health

Chapter One- What I learned on my way back to health

Part Two- How our nation's health got where it is today

Chapter Two- Current population-based health numbers and trends in the United States

Chapter Three- US nutrition trends from World War II to present and some corrective measures we should be taking

Chapter Four- The role of federal government policies on US nutrition trends since the 1970s

Chapter Five- The US Government's current advice on balancing calories consumed against calories expended to control weight in a healthy range does not work

Foreword

"Nothing in biology makes sense except in the light of evolution."
Theodosius Dobzhansky (1900-1975), world-renowned geneticist
and evolutionary biologist.

Taking an evolution-inspired strategy toward nutrition and health
can enhance your life. Our basic DNA programming should drive
how we nourish our bodies; how we move and exercise to stay fit;
how we relate to the world and the people around us; and how we
rest and recover our best selves each day. Evolution should be our
guiding idea, not marketing. We ignore this basic principle at our
peril.

We are the direct descendents of our pre-agricultural ancestors of
10,000 years ago who lived much simpler lives than we do. Their
ancestors lived, thrived and slowly evolved during the millions of
years before widespread agriculture. Evolution gradually shaped
who they became and who we are.

How did they live? They ate what they could find in nature. They
learned to hunt and gather food nearby. In the process, they moved
and "exercised" their bodies. They rested when they were tired.
They had strong social connections that supported them at each
stage of life. Their survival depended on these activities and their
connections to others. They were marvelously healthy compared to
modern Americans.

With the invention of large-scale agriculture, human civilization
made enormous strides forward, but this great gift came with a
price. We moved away from the real whole food our ancient
ancestors consumed. Now, processed food of unimaginable variety
makes up most of the food we consume. Our health has suffered.

General health deterioration in the United States has become
apparent over the last few generations. Obesity is a major problem.
Our health has deteriorated in spite of exceptional progress in
medical science. Chronic diseases are epidemic across our country
and are now spreading throughout the world. These diseases were
virtually unknown to our pre-agricultural ancestors.

Some pressing questions: What is causing these diseases? Are they inevitable as we age? Is poor nutrition to blame? Can the chronic "diseases of civilization," so pervasive in Western countries, be prevented through lifestyle changes?

Evolution Health explores these questions and surveys the most up to date scientific thinking and research on these topics. This book does not promote gimmicks or hype, but relies on solid science supporting potential solutions. You probably will be surprised by some of the concepts raised, although many have been hiding in plain sight.

Evolution Health is a guide to existing information to help you and your family live healthier lives. The information in this book quickly and dramatically turned my health around when I applied it to my own life. I have the medical data to prove it.

Introduction: Part One

Over the last several generations our nation's health has taken an obvious and dramatic turn for the worse. The statistics are overwhelming and sad. Overwhelming in the magnitude of the growing problem and sad in the extensive toll taken on everyday Americans. The toll includes disabilities, debilitating diseases, degraded quality of life and loss of life itself for many people.

And, even worse, the trends in our country are now being repeated around the world as worldwide nutrition patterns come more in line with American food production, distribution and marketing practices. Our food production, distribution and marketing techniques are being exported to more and more countries around the world where the negative health impacts we have experienced are now being repeated.

Only a few generations ago, Americans were relatively healthy. Our pre-agricultural ancestors were even healthier. So, two questions come to mind- why did this downturn in health happen and why does it seem to be escalating now? The causes are multiple, some relatively straight forward and others more elusive. The good news is that a growing body of scientifically valid evidence sheds light on the presumptive causes of our collective ill health and researchers are developing plausible solutions. We will explore this evidence together and I will draw your attention to some practical solutions that have the potential to enhance your health and wellness.

A key part of our problem today can be illuminated by the story of the Tower of Babel. In that story, the residents of Babel decided to build a great city and a tower to heaven. As punishment for their arrogance, God destroyed the tower and the population was splintered forever when the people could no longer communicate with each other. Hence, the word Babel now describes unintelligible speech. We have taken a similar path with our health. Our search was not heavenward but driven by our belief in the power of science. Unfortunately, not all of the science we have been relying upon was grounded in good practice and the advice that flowed from poor scientific practices was frequently flawed.

We live in a Tower of Babel world today. A Google® search in July 2014 of the phrase "diet books" yielded 159 million results in .33 seconds! That is Babel on steroids. It is almost impossible to sort through the countless nutrition, exercise and diet claims and counter-claims and make any sense of the situation by yourself. The relentless marketing of the latest and greatest diets is big business through books, magazines, TV, the Internet and other media channels. Almost every day a celebrity bears her or his soul about how she or he turned things around, lost weight and got a great movie deal by following a "revolutionary" diet. Conveniently their book is now available @Amazon®. Or a doctor recounts how he or she saved his or her patients by designing and prescribing a diet no one ever heard of before. Book also conveniently available @Amazon®. We rarely hear about the long-term success of these amazing diet plans, just the marketing claims and most of these books end up in the recycle bin.

Despite this flood of information, the health trends that matter in our country are getting worse every day, as our own government has meticulously documented. The good news is that together we can discover from the best available scientific information and our own common sense some practical steps we can take to reclaim our natural healthy selves.

Many current researchers are looking at diet and nutrition with a fresh but actually ancient perspective. This older perspective was lost amongst changing beliefs about diet and health that trace back to events in the nineteen fifties, sixties and seventies. These changing beliefs, driven largely by expert opinion, led to a dramatic shift in US government policy that broke from the generally understood folk wisdom everyone knew up until then. It had always been common sense that excessive sugar and sweets and excessive consumption of highly refined grain, especially white wheat flour, and other carbohydrates were probably the main culprits in weight gain and the other medical conditions that seemed to tag along with being significantly overweight. That common sense was lost in the 1970s, for reasons we will explore, but is making a strong comeback with mounting scientific research into our past combined with cutting edge science leading us in a positive direction.

My aim is to act as your guide to these developments and shine additional light on these important events. As I learned in business, you can never communicate too much. Repetition of good ideas is essential to penetrate the general noise and confusion we all experience. This book is one among many telling the important story of how our country got off track on nutrition and health and what can be done to reclaim our natural healthy selves. I want to cut through the confusing deluge of information that exists and point you toward some resources so that you don't have to duplicate the full-time research I have done over a period of many months during my search to get healthier. The information I learned overturned many beliefs I held and, most importantly, when I put it to use transformed my health, as I will describe below. My hope is that it may help you also.

The information and research I will highlight is not my original work. The difficulty has been that it is scattered among many sources, until this book. Because the information is contained in so many places it has been difficult to see a constructive pattern. It has been especially difficult to see a useful pattern that was hidden amongst the Babel of conflicting nutrition claims and counter claims. I will synthesize the information I learned and act as an honest evaluator of the nutrition and exercise claims being presented. I will measure the science behind them against a reasonable standard of proof.

Introduction: Part Two

What is your personal standard of proof necessary to move you to take a new approach toward the food you routinely consume and the way you approach other critical factors affecting your health and wellness? Part of the challenge is that we will never have perfect proof of wellness, nutrition or exercise claims and we don't live in a one size fits all world. What works for some may not work for you. But it helps to have a guiding concept when considering change in your life.

How convincing is the science behind a new idea? The difficulty is that it is virtually impossible to conduct "gold standard" western research studies in the areas of wellness, nutrition and exercise. Controlled, double blind, randomized studies are typically unworkable because of time, expense and compliance (the human element) and causation issues. But we can make some educated choices once we understand the most up to date research even though it may not meet the "gold standard" and apply our own common sense to this wealth of growing information. I want to be your guide to help you easily access the resources I have found that have helped me and that have the potential to help you.

This book is not a breakthrough presenting "new and improved" information. Most of the content was derived from already existing work, some going back decades or more. I did not originally generate the research that serves as the backbone of this book. Other writers and researchers have already done that important work for us. What has been missing until now is a succinct guide to this large and scattered body of information. That is the contribution I hope to make.

My intent is to synthesize the overwhelming amount of existing information and make it more accessible for you, the busy reader. And I hope this book will serve as a real world guide that will help you develop a roadmap for personal action.

Introduction: Part Three

My primary goal is to help spread the word to a wider audience about a growing body of scientifically valid information on human nutrition, exercise and health. The accumulation and dissemination of this knowledge is incredibly dynamic and does not proceed in a straight line. In fact, as Gary Taubes brilliantly described in his encyclopedic book *Good Calories, Bad Calories* (2007) the story is more like a mystery with twists, turns, hidden agendas and surprise discoveries. The real story is actually a lot closer to a John Grisham novel than a dispassionate search for scientific truth.

Taubes shows that valid nutrition advice has been hampered by erroneous belief systems that are remarkably resistant to new discoveries. As he chronicles, these belief systems were usually generated by strong personalities and are now sustained by governmental bureaucratic inertia, economic interests and the inherent limitations of nutrition research. In other words, the human drama playing out in the real world of scientific discovery about human nutrition as it intersects with politics and commerce. This is a very busy intersection!

My second and third goals are to gently urge people in the direction of taking charge of their own nutrition and healthcare, respectively, through some common sense steps.

Fourth, I hope to begin to move the food landscape in our country (and perhaps around the world) in a more positive direction by marshalling the considerable power at our command — the power of consumer spending.

Finally, for those of an activist bent, I have some thoughts based on my professional experience about how we might influence US government policy to build a healthier future for all of us.

At this point you are probably wondering: what are my credentials for this project and how do I propose to do this? Both, very fair questions.

First, I would contend that being overly deferential to credentialed experts (and celebrities) might be part of the problem. We have handed over our health and wellness to credentialed medical and nutrition professionals for at least the last 50 years. Judged by the results, it is fair to say, this has not been an effective strategy. I am not suggesting that credentialed healthcare and nutrition professionals should be ignored — far from it. We need to make these professionals our partners in reclaiming our health. Because health and wellness are our most precious assets, it is worth the time and effort to find out what we can do to optimize them. I think we all would agree, a healthier person has a better chance for a happy and productive life than one coping with disabling medical conditions.

Second, my "credentials" consist of a science and engineering-based education in college (with distinction) at the US Naval Academy in Annapolis where I learned the basics of the scientific method. Generally speaking, the scientific method relies on constructing hypotheses to explain observable attributes of our physical world and testing these hypotheses against the available evidence or through reproducible experiments to confirm or deny the validity of the hypothetical explanation. There are different levels of proof available in science, actually a hierarchy of proofs with different levels of reliability. Sometimes nutrition researchers can carry out well-designed clinical trials to test hypotheses but such gold-standard research is frequently too expensive or possibly unethical or both. Other lesser orders of proof such as observational or epidemiological studies or more loosely controlled but well designed clinical studies can be useful and relied upon to guide us. Even as non-scientists we can be informed by the scientific model to evaluate the health claims made regarding certain human behaviors (both healthy and not so healthy) and draw helpful conclusions. Also, we should trust our common sense in these matters.

Similarly, engineering strives to answer the key question — will a proposed solution work? The chief purpose of engineering is to achieve a desired practical result in the physical world as judged by functionality, safety, reliability, sustainability and cost/benefit, among other things. These same evaluative factors should drive our health and wellness decisions. Does the solution work? Is it safe? What are the risks? Can I stay with it over the long-term? How much does it cost relative to the alternatives? Are there trade-offs involved?

Third, I obtained a law degree (JD with honors) where I learned to read with discernment; and to collect and weigh evidence supporting or refuting a proposition or conclusion. This is one form of critical thinking applied to practical problems. I used this skill every day for over 30 years in my professional endeavors variously as a trial attorney, a regulatory lawyer and a government relations and legal compliance expert. I believe we should apply this same intellectual rigor to the many health, wellness, diet and exercise claims swirling around us. If convincing evidence supports a proposition, we may want to consider putting the proposition to work for us in our daily lives. On the other hand, if a proposition lacks solid evidence we should be leery of acting on it. Is it a real potential solution or just another passing fad? Just as important, who is giving the advice and for what purpose? Is there a hidden motive or agenda behind the advice? Is the advice (or service or product) in my best interests or someone else's?

Fourth, I obtained a second law degree (LLM with honors) that allowed me to move into a 25-year career in healthcare delivery, law and government relations. I worked closely with the elected officials and government agencies that largely shape our healthcare system. I learned how to, and on occasion, actually did influence government policy. I want to put that experience to use, with your help, in shaping a healthier future.

During my career in healthcare, I saw first hand how our healthcare system **spent billions (actually trillions) treating the symptoms** of chronic diseases but very little on prevention. Existing disease prevention, health promotion and "wellness" programs were generally not helping people as promised. These established programs failed to deliver the desired results. I began to wonder why. This led to a personal search for answers that I will briefly describe next and more fully in Chapter One.

Introduction: Part Four

What I learned during my search surprised me and overturned many of the "truths" I had been led to believe during my lifetime. I kept an open mind and tried to find the most scientifically valid approaches to disease prevention, health promotion and wellness. I discovered that the way back to optimum health is not as mystifying as we have been led to believe. The basic answers have been generally understood for many years but for a host of reasons, these common sense lessons from our past became obscured. This book will explore some of the reasons why this happened and where we are today.

As I said earlier, one of the most significant of reasons we have lost our way is the tidal wave of food marketing claims we experience every day many of which are designed to boost sales without regard to health impacts. A second is misguided government policies and their impact on food production, distribution and marketing. Third is the general confusion about how to achieve a healthy life through good nutrition and exercise caused by the Babel of information that can overwhelm us and tends to change every other week. Remember my Google® search results.

The good news is we can relearn the common sense behaviors and folk wisdom our grandparents and ancient ancestors knew that have the potential to restore optimal health. A growing body of scientific research is validating these old obscured truths.

There is an urgent need to begin making better decisions about our health. If we fail to act, our healthcare crisis will only worsen as we chase the latest fad promoted by the latest diet or exercise book only to end up worse off than before we started. Also, continuing to do the same thing that caused the current situation cannot possibly lead to better results (as the popular media frequently reminds us while pitching their preferred solutions).

I want to make some very clear points up front. **I am not a medical doctor. I am not a trained nutritionist or dietician. This is not a diet book. It is a guidebook to existing resources that I believe is worth your consideration.** We don't need anymore scientifically sketchy or ill-conceived diet advice to add to the existing confusion. Even though I am not a medical doctor or a formally trained nutrition expert, what I have learned is based on solid research skills and the application of common sense to the best available information. And as I describe in Chapter One, this information worked for me when I applied it in my own life.

I heard the famous science fiction writer, Robert Heinlein make the following quip at our alma mater, the United States Naval Academy in Annapolis in the early 1970s. He said: "Ninety percent of all Science Fiction is trash – ninety percent of anything is trash." In my view, the ratio is even worse for diet, nutrition and exercise advice coming through popular media. We need to heed the scientifically valid advice and discard the trash. That's where this book comes in. I will introduce you to some nutrition (and exercise) resources that get it mostly right based on reliable evidence, not hype. I will provide a survey of some of these sources and synthesize the lessons in a useful way.

These sources don't agree on every detail but there is remarkable consistency on the main conclusions and the path we need to take to reclaim our health and wellness. These books have been written by diverse authors willing to go back and re-examine the evidence behind our beliefs about healthy nutrition and exercise. They rely on and catalogue a rapidly growing body of scientifically valid nutrition research from around the world. Some of these authors also explain how nutrition policy in the United States dramatically changed in the 1970s as it became detached from the common sense, science-based principles that comprised what "everyone knew" up until then. To our detriment, US government nutrition policies became politically and economically driven to an unfortunate degree and American citizens are now paying the price for these decisions. We will explore these developments together.

I believe this book will provide valid information that can help you and your family members get healthier, but only if you act on it.

Please understand there are no quick fixes or magic bullets (or pills or potions) that will solve our country's healthcare crisis or improve our personal wellness. But if we begin to understand and apply some common sense concepts informed by the best scientific evidence available today in our daily lives, we can begin to make progress.

Ed Cotter
Scottsdale, Arizona

Part One- My personal journey back to health

Chapter One- What I learned on my way back to health.

My food consumption was fairly typical for an American of my generation. I was born in 1951. I ate what I thought was a reasonably good diet according to "what everyone knew." As I got into my early 40s, I developed high blood pressure and my blood biochemistry became problematic. My healthcare providers reassured me that this process was a normal consequence of getting older and that pills would take care of the problem if it got worse. I worked a high stress job for many years as a Navy lawyer and then after I retired from the Navy in 1993, as a corporate regulatory lawyer and compliance and government relations expert for some very large healthcare companies.

I had a real health scare early in 2005 brought on by work-related stress, (undiagnosed) high blood pressure (BP) and an underlying (undiagnosed) condition in my brain. Technically the problem is called a cryptic arterial ventricular malformation or cryptic AVM. That existing condition in combination with high BP led to a minor stroke. I spent 5 miserable days in ICU. The EMTs, doctors, nurses and other healthcare workers saved my life. For that, I am ever grateful. Statistically, I could have died but was lucky to have no lasting impacts other than a lifetime prescription to BP medicines. When my internal medicine specialist told me to find a general practitioner to take over my care in 2006 he said I needed to "eat better and get more exercise." Needless to say, that non-specific advice didn't help much. I kept doing what I had done before eating a "balanced" diet high in refined grains, some sugar and lots of salty snacks. I knew the salty snacks were not healthy but I rationalized that otherwise I ate a healthy diet and overall things were "in balance." I was wrong.

I got a decent amount of exercise over the years although

exercise frequently took a back seat to my demanding work schedule. I ate food based on what I had absorbed from the culture and what was readily available. What I had absorbed was, unfortunately, a jumble of conflicting information, not all of it sound. Much of my food consumption was driven by our food production, marketing and distribution systems including such seemingly mundane factors as product placement in grocery stores, discount coupons, special pricing and other forms of marketing. Government advice in the form of the food pyramid and other government pronouncements about a "balanced" diet with lots of "healthy grains" also informed my opinions. Its easy to convince ourselves that chowing down at the Olive Garden (or any similar eatery) was following the healthy "Mediterranean diet" as long as you throw in a side salad.

I had always been athletic so my weight was not a major problem although it continued to go up slowly after I retired from the Navy at age 41. My waistline expanded gradually also. Again, I was reassured that these changes were the normal consequences of growing older. My heaviest point was around 200 pounds in the 2008-12 timeframe. I am just under 6 feet tall so I was a just a bit overweight by conventional standards. My medical professionals never made my weight an issue during annual check-ups, in fact, I was usually complemented for being in good shape, **for my age,** implying that getting fatter was just a natural consequence of getting older.

Early in 2013 I started to look into the connection between diet, exercise and wellness because my standard cardio workouts had only lowered my weight from 200 to 193 and my blood biochemistry was not ideal. I was taking 4 BP meds per day and wanted to find a better way. I read everything I could lay my hands on and became convinced that a Paleo approach might help me achieve my health and wellness goals.

Paleo nutrition is based on the concept that we are biologically no different from our Paleolithic ancestors and that many of our modern health problems can be remedied by going back to a nutrition pattern similar to what Paleolithic hunter-gatherers (and their modern equivalents) consumed. This approach was popularized by Loren Cordain, PhD in his book *The Paleo Diet* (2002 hardcover, 2011 paperback) and the popular follow-on *The Paleo Solution* by Robb Wolf (2010). Paleo nutrition has been **mocked as the Caveman diet** but the scientific evidence behind it is quite convincing, at least to me. Dr. Cordain has documented the considerable science behind his recommendations based on a 30-year academic career studying the subject. The Paleo hypothesis follows from two established facts. First, our genetic make-up is virtually the same as our ancient Paleolithic ancestors. Second, our current diet is radically different from what they ate. I became convinced that this mismatch might be my problem. I decided to pattern my food intake in a way driven by what my body really needed for optimal health and not by marketing claims and government policy. In essence, I conducted a nutritional experiment on myself to test the Paleo hypothesis as developed by Dr. Cordain and refined by his acolyte, Robb Wolf.

I made significant changes to my nutrition starting August 1, 2013 and eliminated processed food and added sugar from my diet. I was following a Paleo approach but was concerned about the rigidity of the diet and whether I could stick with it. As I have learned subsequently, maintaining a healthy diet is the most important factor in long-term success. Starting a new diet is relatively easy, as is some early weight loss, but long-term successful maintenance of the early gains is not. I was highly motivated to make the changes but wondered how long I could stay away from certain off-limits foods that make up the bulk of our modern diets. Another concern was that Paleo would be too boring. I found some excellent Paleo cookbooks that addressed this concern. These cookbooks are listed in Appendix B. The cookbooks gave my family and me a number of good ideas. We eat a more varied and delicious diet than ever these days.

I found *The Primal Blueprint* by Mark Sisson (2009 hardcover, 2012 paperback) two weeks into my Paleo experiment and read it cover to cover very quickly. Primal is a variation on the

Paleo approach. I liked the flexibility of Mark' Sisson's 80/20 rule and the idea that Primal is not about perfection or ideology but about enjoying life and getting healthier. The 80/20 rule allows for occasional non-Primal foods but encourages greater adherence to the *Primal Blueprint* over time. As a probable Type A personality, I had already subjected my body to a lot of stress over the years and did not want to repeat that mistake by trying to follow a rigid diet down to the letter. Based on Mark's book and the supportive information on Marksdailyapple.com I modified my nutrition to the more flexible Primal way. It was a great fit for me and I have stayed with it ever since.

The results were dramatic. I started losing weight very quickly in the first few weeks. That tapered off after about 2 months but continued on a nice glide path over the next 4 months. At 6 months my weight was down to 168 pounds, the same as when I graduated from college in 1973!

I feel I have probably added 8-10 pounds of muscle doing Primal workouts that feature shorter more intense strength routines so that is a total of 30+ pounds of useless fat gone. Actually it is not just useless fat, as I will discuss later. I've added my own flourishes to Mark's Primal exercise approach and really enjoy working out again. I throw in some short intense interval sprint work on the elliptical from time to time but not the old boring cardio stuff that drained my energy. I do as much walking and hiking as I can. When I started my strength workouts I had trouble doing one pull-up. Now I can do 12. I can also do 50 push-ups. A current photo is next that shows the positive results overall.

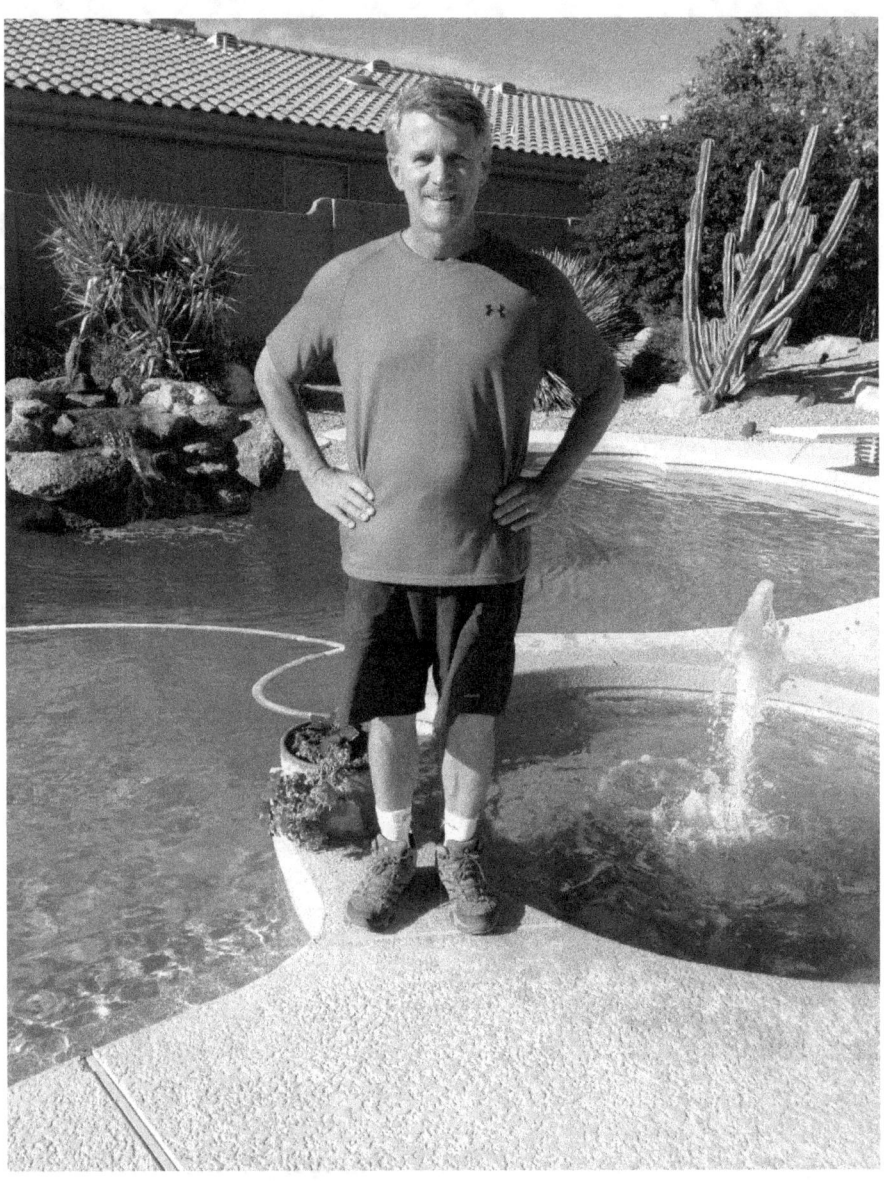

One of my primary goals was to shed the slab of fat around my belly button. I have learned that a "spare tire" is not just an aesthetic concern but also a significant health risk because of the unhealthy hormonal changes this store of visceral fat brings with it. Visceral fat is an active hormone factory that disrupts our entire hormonal system and over time can lead to chronic illnesses like type 2 diabetes, heart disease and even cancer.

Right away my waist began to noticeably shrink. I liked that and was very motivated to stay the course. My waist went from 39+ down to 32.5 over 9 months.

A totally unexpected positive happened: my hair got darker!

There was one "downside." I had to get my pants taken in because they no longer fit.

My problematic blood profile improved dramatically in just 6 weeks to the amazement of my healthcare professional. *She wanted me to tell her how I did it, which I was happy to do*! I only take 2 BP meds per day now and hope to wean off them someday.

My current triglycerides to HDL cholesterol ratio is 0.93 down from dangerous levels just 2 years ago. This ratio is a key indicator of heart health and is closely correlated with the risk of heart attack. The consensus in medical circles is that anything below 2.0 is healthy. The ratio is easy to derive from a basic panel of blood work: just divide the triglycerides number by the HDL cholesterol number.

I am grateful I have been able to improve my health and intend to stay with a Primal approach for the rest of my life. Almost two years later I am still with it. Some of my family members and friends have also gotten positive results from eating more real, whole food and generally skipping the processed stuff. This is the essence of *eating like a caveman*. This nutrition pattern is actually closer to the way our grandparents ate just a few generations ago. Some have dismissed Paleo/Primal nutrition as unsound, possibly even unhealthy, but it has worked for me and many thousands of people. I have the lab numbers to prove I am healthier now.

I want others to enjoy the health improving results I have been able to achieve. How? First, people need specific scientifically validated nutrition information presented in a concise manner. Second, to get the positive results people need to apply this information to their daily routines. Third, people need to be able to stick with it over the long-term or else the early gains will quickly disappear. This is the problem illustrated by yo-yo dieting.

The primary goal of this book is to spread the word about the nutrition and exercise information I have learned and help people who are willing to make some changes in their lives to recapture or preserve their health.

Note: a slightly different version of my story was posted October 10, 2014 as a regular Friday feature of Primal Success Stories on the popular website — Marksdailyapple.com. The site is run by Mark Sisson the author of *The Primal Blueprint* and is dedicated to all aspects of Primal living. Primal living is a variation on the Paleo lifestyle. The website is free but it is a vehicle to market products.

Part Two- How our nation's health got where it is today.

Chapter Two- Current population-based health numbers and trends in the United States.

> "The most recent data indicate that 72 percent of men and 64 percent of women are overweight or obese, with about one-third of adults being obese. Even in the absence of overweight, poor diet and physical inactivity are associated with major causes of morbidity and mortality. These include cardiovascular disease, hypertension, type 2 diabetes, osteoporosis, and some types of cancer." *Dietary Guidelines for Americans 2010* pgs. 9-10.

> "As a nation [the United States], more than 75% of our health care spending is on people with chronic conditions. These persistent conditions—the nation's leading causes of death and disability—leave in their wake deaths that could have been prevented, lifelong disability, compromised quality of life, and burgeoning health care costs." *The Power of Prevention, Chronic disease . . . the public health Challenge of the 21st Century-* a report by the Center for Disease Control and Prevention (CDC), US Department of Health and Human Services (DHHS) (2009)

... our health care system is not designed to prevent chronic illnesses."
Id.

Researchers estimate that the 2014 cost of treating preventable chronic diseases in the United States will exceed $2 trillion. YES, TWO TRILLION DOLLARS IN ONE YEAR! The amount is literally incomprehensible. The challenge is both financial and, in my view, moral. Is this the best use of our precious resources? Is there nothing we can do to slow, halt or reverse these alarming health trends and reduce the projected expenditures? Do we have the will and the spirit to do it? What kind of future do we want to bequeath to our children and grand children? These are questions that require serious reflection and action, I believe.

The current health numbers are ominous. No informed source disputes this starting point. Lets review some of the statistics from federal government sources to put the situation in perspective.

The data below comes directly from the *Dietary Guidelines for Americans 2010* page 16. This report provides the official position of our government on proper nutrition and other lifestyle choices and has an enormous impact on food production and consumption patterns in the United States. Here is their status report on the current state of our health (with footnotes omitted):

"The heavy toll of diet-related chronic diseases

cardiovascular disease
• 81.1 million Americans—37 percent of the population—have cardiovascular disease. Major risk factors include high levels of blood cholesterol and other lipids, type 2 diabetes, hypertension (high blood pressure), metabolic syndrome, overweight and obesity, physical inactivity, and tobacco use.
• 16 percent of the U.S. adult population has high total blood cholesterol.

hypertension
• 74.5 million Americans—34 percent of U.S. adults—have hypertension.
• Hypertension is a major risk factor for heart disease, stroke, congestive heart failure, and kidney disease.
• Dietary factors that increase blood pressure include excessive sodium and insufficient potassium intake, overweight and obesity, and excess alcohol consumption.

• 36 percent of American adults have prehypertension—blood pressure numbers that are higher than normal, but not yet in the hypertension range.

diabetes

• Nearly 24 million people—almost 11 percent of the population—ages 20 years and older have diabetes. The vast majority of cases are type 2 diabetes, which is heavily influenced by diet and physical activity.

• About 78 million Americans—35 percent of the U.S. adult population ages 20 years or older—have pre-diabetes. Pre-diabetes (also called impaired glucose tolerance or impaired fasting glucose) means that blood glucose levels are higher than normal, but not high enough to be called diabetes.

cancer

• Almost one in two men and women—approximately 41 percent of the population—will be diagnosed with cancer during their lifetime.

• Dietary factors are associated with risk of some types of cancer, including breast (post- menopausal), endometrial, colon, kidney, mouth, pharynx, larynx, and esophagus.

osteoporosis

• One out of every two women and one in four men ages 50 years and older will have an osteoporosis-related fracture in their lifetime.

• About 85 to 90 percent of adult bone mass is acquired by the age of 18 in girls and the age of 20 in boys. Adequate nutrition and regular participation in physical activity are important factors in achieving and maintaining optimal bone mass."

Above is the 2010 snapshot. What are the trends? Are Americans getting healthier or sicker?

The LA times reported on June 22, 2015 that: "Americans have reached a weighty milestone: Adults who are obese now outnumber those who are merely overweight, according to a new report in the journal JAMA Internal Medicine."

Data reported in a July 23, 2014 article summarizing the findings of a Johns Hopkins Bloomberg School of Public Health study of extensive Medicare claims data speaks to the trends effecting older Americans.

"With nearly four in five older Americans living with multiple chronic medical conditions, a new study by researchers at Johns Hopkins Bloomberg School of Public Health finds that the more ailments you have after retirement age, the shorter your life expectancy.

"The analysis, one of the first to examine the burden of multiple chronic conditions on life expectancy among the elderly, may help explain why increases in life expectancy among older Americans are slowing. [Emphasis added]

"A report on the findings, based on an analysis of 1.4 million Medicare enrollees, appears in the August 2014 issue of the journal *Medical Care.*

> ""Living with multiple chronic diseases such as diabetes, kidney disease and heart failure is now the norm and not the exception in the United States," says Eva H. DuGoff, a recent PhD recipient at the Johns Hopkins Bloomberg School of Public Health and lead author of the report. "The medical advances that have allowed sick people to live longer may not be able to keep up with the growing burden of chronic disease. **It is becoming very clear that <u>preventing</u> the development of additional chronic conditions in the elderly could be the <u>only way</u> to continue to improve life expectancy.**" [Emphasis added]

We have been using all of the modern tools of medical practice to treat these chronic conditions. Applying some of that energy and those resources to preventing chronic diseases before they strike is worth trying. Continuing on the path we are currently moving along will not solve the problem, as this report suggests. The report very clearly recommends a more robust prevention strategy.

These are not esoteric issues and this is not an academic debate. The real world consequences of our current approach are all around us. The problems are so pervasive that virtually every family in the United States is being affected, often in tragic ways, but most certainly in degraded quality of life for one or more loved ones. The situation does not have to continue. These trends are not inevitable. With the right knowledge and some commitment to making healthier decisions our future can be improved. At least I hope so.

Chapter Three- US nutrition trends from World War II to present and some corrective measures we should be taking.

We know that World War II (WWII) had significant impact on food consumption in the United States. The impact was even more extreme in other parts of the world that became actual battlegrounds. One impact in the US was that sugar was rationed and therefore daily consumption was restricted below the amounts people would have consumed if sugar had been more readily available. As I will discuss later, sugar consumption has grown rapidly since this period of reduced availability and many experts believe it now poses a substantial threat to our nation's health. In addition, a new sweetening substance called High Fructose Corn Syrup (HFCS) was introduced into the American food supply in the late 1970s and it use has grown dramatically ever since.

You may be aware of Robert Lustig, MD's excellent video *Sugar- The Bitter Truth* (2009) available on YouTube® that lays out a clear medical case against the copious amounts of sugar (fructose) ingested annually by Americans. He traces the alarming rise in average sugar consumption since WWII focusing on the disastrous impact this is having on children, his medical specialty. Per capita consumption of fructose, the most problematic chemical in sugar, HFCS and processed fruit juice stands at 141 pounds per year. Other sources calculate even higher consumption figures. It is important to understand, and as the video makes clear, processed fruit juice is really just another sugary drink with limited nutritional value once it has gone through processing. In plain language, processed fruit juice is no healthier than other sugary drinks. This came as a surprise to me in my research because I had always thought that my favorite orange juice was a great way to get a healthy start to the day. The reality is this large dose of fructose first thing in the morning sets you up for some unhealthy hormonal ups and downs that take a toll on the body over time. The video explains the medical science behind Dr. Lustig's conclusion that "sugar [fructose] is toxic" to the human body.

Note that table sugar (sucrose) is 50% fructose and 50% glucose and HFCS is 55% fructose and 45% glucose. They are virtually identical chemicals when processed in the human body. Not only does excess sugar cause us to get fat, it brings along many other related health problems over the longer term, especially type 2 diabetes and heart disease. This may seem surprising because sugar looks clean and tastes good — how can sugar cause health problems? Lustig makes a compelling and surprising case that a regular (non-diet) soda is the same as a beer once consumed because alcohol and sugar look and act the same chemically in the human body. He asks pointedly, would you serve your young child a can of beer? Dr. Lustig followed up on *Sugar- The Bitter Truth* with *Fat Chance: Fructose 2.0* in 2013 where he urges all of us to take a more active role in reversing the troubling trends in sugar consumption in the United States, especially among the young.

Our federal government's official nutrition advice contained in the *Dietary Guidelines for Americans 2010* gets this point right and recommends reduced sugar consumption. Unfortunately, this key point tends to get lost in the lengthy government report. Also, this important part of the government's message competes with and tends to lose out against other forces shaping consumer behavior. These other stronger counter-influences are at work moving sugar consumption trends in the wrong direction. Dr. Lustig traces this countertrend, in part, to government decisions made in the 1970s to increase monetary subsidies for sugar production. What we have is different parts of the federal government working in opposite directions. One part urges us to consume less sugar and the other provides monetary subsidies that increase sugar production and consumption.

Economic theory tells us there will be more of an activity when the activity is subsidized (i.e. paid for by the government or someone else). That is exactly what happened and continues to happen today as American consumers do not have to pay the real cost of the sugar they consume. Cheaper sugar means more sugar consumed. There is nothing mysterious about this predictable cause and effect. Refined sugar and its cousin,

HFCS, are in almost every processed food made today. Dr. Lustig estimates that 80% of all processed foods contain added sugar. Sweet drinks of almost infinite variety are loaded with sugar and HFCS. These sweetened drinks and processed foods are a huge and growing business and younger Americans are the biggest consumers. As mentioned earlier, processed fruit juices, marketed as a healthy alternative, are really not much different from sugary drinks like soda and "sports" drinks. The marketing and advertising of these products involves multi-million dollar investments every year by some of the most iconic brands in the world. Clearly, the companies know what they are doing to increase sales. It's good for their businesses but we should ask ourselves if it is good for us.

I want to stress here that I am a strong proponent of business, especially American business. Responsible free enterprise and general economic freedom have done more to help more people achieve the "good life" than any other system yet invented. The system of free choice and voluntary exchange brings a profusion of products to market. Our lives are richer as a result. Our robust business environment has brought many benefits to our country, to many people around the world and to me personally. I have started businesses and helped build others within corporate environments. I'm proud of those actions. That said, the impact of any business transaction on our society — positive or negative — is fair game for examination. I believe that as consumers we need to consider the overall impact of a business transaction when we buy a product or service. Whether a product is health promoting or not should be an important consideration, especially when it comes to the food we eat.

A second major nutrition trend in the US is the increasing consumption of refined carbohydrates (other than sugar). The proliferation of highly refined carbohydrates, primarily wheat milled into flour, has been chronicled in the best selling diet book *Wheat Belly* by William Davis, MD (2011 hardcover, 2014 paperback). Dr. Davis describes in his witty style how wheat has come to dominate the American diet and his belief about the unhealthful consequences of this major shift. He states

"Wheat as a crop has succeeded on an unprecedented scale.... It is by a long stretch, among the most consumed grains on earth, constituting 20 percent of all calories consumed." *Wheat Belly* at pg. 13. OK, so is this a problem?

Dr. Davis makes the observation that wheat is a substance that has many natural defenses against consumption. These defenses are the built-in means to ensure wheat's survival against other living species. Without these natural defenses wheat would have lost out in the evolutionary competition over time. In addition, and even more significantly, modern wheat is radically different from wheat that was used to make bread since the beginning of agriculture until recently. Now, highly sophisticated gene-modifying techniques are used to create high-yield wheat with different properties. In one fascinating chapter Dr. Davis details how the wheat in our modern diet is not at all similar to the wheat of 50, 150 or 2,000 years ago and he describes why this new modern wheat is a threat to our health. *Wheat Belly* at Chapter 2. He makes a strong case that the natural protections against wheat consumption that have always been contained in wild wheat combined with the recent genetic modifications in modern wheat have made this food even more incompatible with human consumption than ever. He argues that we are in a period where wheat consumption is one of the most significant causes of growing human obesity and obesity's associated chronic diseases (among other adverse health consequences).

He recommends the **elimination of wheat** in all its processed forms as the prescription for reclaiming health and wellness. He also recommends drastically reducing current excessive sugar consumption that, not coincidentally, is contained in many of the same processed foods made primarily with refined wheat. The sweeteners are added for the simple reason that highly processed grain does not taste good by itself. Just add some sugar and salt and, presto, you have a tasty snack. The result is an astonishing array of snacks, cereals and pastas available at your local grocery store and a similar number of tasty treats in the bakery section. The bad news is these highly processed wheat products are believed to be causing many of the confounding chronic diseases we live with today.

Of course, there are other viewpoints on the topic of wheat. We know that the processed food companies spend lavishly to convince us that their products are healthy. Our government recommends whole wheat as part of the balanced diet. Even universities are in the mix. For example, the March 2014 Tufts University Health and Nutrition Newsletter ran the following lead story: *The Truth About the War on Wheat.* It is easy to discern the position they took from the title. Here is a quote from Nicola McKeown, PhD identified as an associate professor at Tufts and a **scientific advisor to the Whole Wheat Council:** "There is a lack of scientific evidence to support the claims that eating wheat is an independent risk factor for greater abdominal adiposity or weight gain." There are more than a few qualifiers in that sentence but I'm sure we can trust that an advisor to the Whole Wheat Council will give us the truth about wheat consumption.

I am always on guard when people use a "lack of evidence" or the trendy phrase "no evidence" to support a conclusion. These empty phrases logically prove nothing. Common sense tells us that a "lack of scientific evidence" is not evidence that an idea is false, only that the tools of science have not yet confirmed or denied the hypothesis. Another critical caveat in the article is that the authors praise only "whole wheat" and acknowledge that highly processed wheat is a problem by stating "It's true that refined grains including wheat have been stripped of much of their natural nutrition, and that processed carbohydrates — often eaten in the mistaken pursuit of a low-fat diet — have contributed to America's obesity epidemic." So, I am a little confused by the position they advocate. "Whole wheat" is good, but the article acknowledges that most of the wheat products Americans actually eat are nutritionally degraded and are making us fat. In addition they state that the **mistaken** pursuit of a low-fat diet is also part of the problem. In other words, following the government advice to cut fat and eat more whole grains (official federal government policy that I will discuss more fully later) has had the unintended effect of increasing the consumption of nutritionally deficient refined wheat flour that is contributing to the obesity epidemic. Precisely the point argued in *Wheat Belly*. I'm ready to vote on this one. The debate winner is — Dr. Davis.

Wheat Belly advances a viewpoint about the negative effects of refined grain on our midsections and the organs nearby but what about other organs in the human body that may also be damaged by grain consumption?

Enter David Permutter, MD with evidence that modern refined grain is damaging to your brain's health. The #1 NY Times bestseller *Grain Brain* by David Perlmutter, MD with Kristin Loberg (2013)- subtitled "The surprising truth about wheat, carbs and sugar- your brain's silent killers," makes the case that modern refined grain in combination with excessive carbs and sugar are very bad for your brain's health.

Another physician, Suzanne de la Monte, MD, MPH of Brown University has been credited as the first to call Alzheimer's disease "type 3 diabetes." The implications of her research are that the same factors leading to the epidemic of type 2 diabetes in our country are also driving dramatic increases in Alzheimer's. See the *New York Times* online September 25, 2012 article by Mark Bittman.

Dr. Permutter's argument is provocative and many will dismiss his conclusions. But what if he is just earlier to the party than others? The good doctor is a board certified neurologist and a fellow of the American College of Nutrition. He is the only doctor in the country to hold both of these certifications. He has a certified background and 35 years of clinical experience in his corner. His mission is to prevent neurological problems before they happen. I am a firm believer in prevention over treatment. He comes right out swinging with the following statement about the wheat in our current food distribution system: "With modern hybridization and gene-modifying technology, the 133 pounds of wheat that the average American consumes each year shares no genetic, structural or chemical likeness to what hunter-gatherers might have stumbled upon." *Grain Brain* at page 8. In other words, he makes the uncontroversial point that the wheat in our modern processed foods is not the wheat our grandparents ate and bears no resemblance to wheat from the very early agricultural period, not to mention during Paleolithic times. The problem: "We are increasingly challenging our physiology with ingredients for which we are not genetically prepared." *Id.* This is the same logic behind the Paleo diet. This logic suggests that we are not genetically adapted to eat modern processed foods and may never be. Remember that evolution is a very, very slow process. It follows that we cannot thrive on these processed foods as they are currently constituted because they do not provide the essential nutrition our bodies need.

And as Dr. Perlmutter explains, there is a good deal of evidence that these foods are causing real damage to our brains. Our brain is arguably the most important organ in the body and certainly the one that makes us uniquely human. His viewpoint is important and should be considered on the question of whether refined grains should be the mainstay of our diets. He states: "Researchers have known for some time now that the cornerstone of all degenerative conditions, including brain disorders, is inflammation." *Id.* at page 33. "And what they are finding is that gluten, and a high carbohydrate diet for that matter, are among the most prominent stimulators of inflammatory pathways that reach the brain." *Id.* Dr. Perlmutter is a strong proponent of prevention. The pillar of his prevention strategy is the elimination of processed grains from our diets. The reason prevention is so important is straightforward: "When it comes to brain disease, once the diagnosis is in for something like dementia, turning the train around is hard," *Id.*

He also spends time debunking what he calls two popular myths. The myths are that: "... (1) a low fat high carbohydrate diet is good [current US government guidelines], and (2) cholesterol is bad." *Id.* Most of us are aware that we have been fighting a battle against "high" cholesterol for many years, primarily with drug therapy, and mostly losing the fight. I will not attempt to repeat his work here but I recommend his counter-intuitive advice for your consideration. He is not alone in arguing against a pharmaceutical-based approach to managing cholesterol. In fact, he makes the case that cholesterol is not a problem to be managed with drugs but is absolutely necessary for good health and can be optimized by proper nutrition and exercise. As we learn more about the complexities of cholesterol, and there are many, the better science is moving toward a much more nuanced view. We now have a much more helpful approach to interpreting the cholesterol numbers in our lab test results and understanding how the food we consume is driving the numbers in the report.

There is an obvious challenge implementing the recommendations Dr. Davis, Dr. Permutter and many others make to eliminate grains from our diets. The difficulty is the ubiquitous nature of grain in the typical American diet today and the relentless marketing of refined grain based products. It is not easy to go grain-free in our modern world. And to be brutally honest, the vast array of products produced with modern refined grain are really tasty. My personal favorites are all manner of salty crunchy snacks... and they know who they are. It does not help that this advice is also at odds with mainstream nutrition advice from the certified experts and as promulgated by our federal government. More on that in the next chapter.

The personal question we each need to answer becomes — is the short-term pleasure of a grain based diet worth the potential long-term pain?

Chapter Four- The role of federal government policies on US nutrition trends since the 1970s.

Many authors trace the government's active participation in shaping nutrition in the United States to three interwoven events that occurred in the nineteen seventies. The three strands that came together in this decade still largely shape US government nutrition policy today. I will discuss each in this Chapter.

First, and most significantly, was the seminal statement on nutrition by the US Senate Committee headed by George McGovern in 1977 that ultimately led to national nutrition guidelines issued in 1980, the Food Guide Pyramid in 1992, MyPyramid in 2005 and MyPlate in 2011. Second, was an emerging trend in the research that declared that reducing fat in the diet and increasing carbohydrates was the best way to protect heart health. Third was a political intervention in agricultural subsidies that lowered the cost of refined sugar (and later of High Fructose Corn Syrup) sparking a surge in the consumption of these two virtually identical products.

We will explore the role of the McGovern Senate Committee in changing the direction of food consumption in the United States.

According to a US government report issued by the USDA, this important event in our history happened this way:

"In early 1977, after years of discussion, scientific review, and debate, the Senate Select Committee on Nutrition and Human Needs, led by Senator George McGovern, recommended Dietary Goals for the American people. The Committee recommended that the American diet:

- Increase carbohydrate intake to 55 to 60 percent of calories
- Decrease dietary fat intake to no more than 30 percent of calories, with a reduction in intake of saturated fat, and recommended approximately equivalent

distributions among saturated, polyunsaturated, and monounsaturated fats to meet the 30 percent target
- Decrease cholesterol intake to 300 mg per day
- Decrease sugar intake to 15 percent of calories
- Decrease salt intake to 3 g per day

"The issuance of the Dietary Goals was met with a great deal of debate and controversy from both industry groups and the scientific community. These groups believed the science might not have supported the specificity of the numbers in the Dietary Goals. (Emphasis added)

> "To support the credibility of the science used by the Committee, the Department of Agriculture and, at that time, the Department of Health, Education, and Welfare pulled together scientists from the two Departments and expertise from the scientific community throughout the country. In February 1980, the Dietary Guidelines for Americans brochure was issued collaboratively by the two Departments and represented their points of view, at that time, on ways to build a healthful diet and lifestyle."

This sequence of events led directly to the current government nutrition guidelines that are little changed from those issued by the McGovern Committee in 1977. In recent years the criticism of these initial recommendations and the subsequent government recommendations, most recently re-issued in 2010 and discussed more fully below, has not quieted down. Many experts believe the initial goals were not supported by compelling scientific evidence at the time nor are the subsequent guidelines that we live with today. Common sense, our own observations of the state of public health generally and the growing health epidemics of preventable chronic diseases (even by our government's own admission) support this criticism. The evidence should, at the very least, provoke an honest reevaluation of the guidelines that have after a trial of three and one half decades failed to produce the desired health improvements in the US population.

Gary Taubes encyclopedic book *Good Calories, Bad Calories,* Chapter 3 (2007) provides a revealing look behind the scenes at the McGovern Committee's work. He summarizes the situation by saying at page 45 "*Dietary Goals* [the shorthand version of the name] took a grab bag of ambiguous studies and speculation, admitted that the claims were scientifically contentious, and then officially bestowed on one interpretation the aura of fact." Taubes explains that the *Dietary Goals* were written by a former journalist under the advice of an advocate for the nutrition principles that became the *Goals* main themes. In other words, the document was largely political in nature and not a scientific exposition of the state of nutritional research at the time.

No doubt Senator McGovern acted in good faith on a problem he felt was urgent. Senator McGovern was a patriot who flew dangerous bombing missions in Europe during World War II earning a Distinguished Flying Cross for his heroic actions. He was a serious and dedicated politician who believed the government needed to act to head off a growing nutrition crisis. So he took action through his Senate committee. His committee report, later slightly revised to respond to criticism, has driven health policy in the United States to this day. This would be fine if the report and the guidelines had the desired effect and had actually improved health in our country. However, America's health has worsened rather than improved during this time. As criticism has mounted in recent years, it is far past time to take a hard look at our government's nutrition policies and see if a different approach is appropriate.

In addition to issuing the *Dietary Guidelines*, and subsequent pronouncements a second part of the Committee's work was important in shaping nutrition policy and food consumption in the US. This is the second strand of the story.

Throughout the nineteen forties, fifties and sixties a debate raged among professional nutrition researchers about the effect on individual and societal health of consuming certain foods. This debate mainly pitted a dietary fat hypothesis against a refined carbohydrate hypothesis as he main cause of heart disease. Gary Taubes details the ins and outs of the research and debate brilliantly in *Good Calories, Bad Calories*. My interest is not primarily in the debate itself, but in the resolution of the debate and the subsequent impact on government nutrition research funding policy.

Mr. Taubes states that the McGovern report of 1977 was decisive in "settling" the debate in favor of what he calls the "Keys hypothesis." *Good Calories, Bad Calories* at page 44. The Keys hypothesis fell into the dietary fat hypothesis camp. This hypothesis held that dietary fat and dietary cholesterol were causing heart disease and that these foods should be reduced in the American diet. The other side of the hypothesis was that carbohydrate consumption, primarily of refined grains, should be increased. This drove federal nutrition policy. As we now know, this policy represented a triumph of hope over the reality that unfolded.

The Keys reference is to a very influential researcher Ancel Keys who made it onto the cover of Time magazine in January 1961 as a result of his groundbreaking research. Mr. Taubes and others have spent considerable intellectual capital reviewing Ancel Keys research and have found it wanting. Taubes and others have shown that Keys used a subset of the data he and his team collected to support his conclusions while excluding data gathered at the same time that did not support or actually refuted his conclusions. In other words, he selectively picked the data to support a conclusion. This is not good science.

What is clear now is that Keys' early work in nutrition research had a powerful impact on the agencies of the US government that fund nutrition research projects. Taubes notes that after the McGovern report, federal government funding tended to go to researchers who sought to confirm the government's policy as announced in the McGovern Committee's work and later contained in the government's official Guidelines, but not to government policy skeptics. As a result, alternative research was de-funded and "pro-government" research was overfunded. This would not be a problem if the government's conclusions were based on good science and best available research techniques or if we were actually becoming healthier as a result of this government intervention. Unfortunately, that is not what is happening to the health trends that really matter.

The opposite has turned out to be true. And after many years of dedicated, government funded research the case still has not been made that dietary fat, dietary cholesterol and related higher cholesterol measures are causing heart disease. Nor has the documented reduction of dietary fat in the American diet produced the desired results. Government policy has achieved reductions in fat intake and increases in carbohydrate consumption but the expected beneficial results have not followed. As Gary Taubes states "In the decades since the NIH, the surgeon general and the National Academy of Sciences first declared that all Americans should consume low-fat diets, the research has also failed to support the most critical aspect of this recommendation: that such diets will lead to a longer and healthier life. On the contrary, it has consistently indicated that these diets may cause more harm than good." *Good Calories, Bad Calories* at page 80. This is a staggering statement. The government's recommendations have led to a less healthy American population? Sounds like we need to rethink what we have been told and, perhaps, come up with a new plan.

The third strand of this story was the decision by the federal government in the nineteen seventies to increase monetary subsidies to the sugar cane and corn growers to reduce the price of dietary sweeteners and bring more sugar and High Fructose Corn Syrup (HFCS) to the American table. As discussed earlier in highlighting Dr. Robert Lustig's work, the per capita sugar consumption of Americans has grown substantially since World War II and continues to grow. Dr Lustig is so concerned about this trend because as he has stated in his videos "sugar is toxic" to humans. While some may question the choice of words, the evidence grows that excessive sugar consumption is a significant factor in our growing obesity and diabetes problems. Sadly, younger Americans are being adversely affected by this trend as much or more than other age groups. They develop a taste for sweet products early in life and the harmful consequences follow from lifelong over-consumption.

Chapter Five- The US Government's current advice on balancing calories consumed against calories expended to control weight in a healthy range does not work!

> "Achieving and sustaining appropriate body weight across the lifespan is vital to maintaining good health and quality of life. Many behavioral, environmental, and genetic factors have been shown to affect a person's body weight. **Calorie balance over time is the key to weight management.** Calorie balance refers to the relationship between calories consumed from foods and beverages and calories expended in normal body functions (i.e., metabolic processes) and through physical activity. People cannot control the calories expended in metabolic processes, but they can control what they eat and drink, as well as how many calories they use in physical activity. "Calories consumed must equal calories expended for a person to maintain the same body weight. Consuming more calories than expended will result in weight gain. **Conversely, consuming fewer calories than expended will result in weight loss. This can be achieved over time by eating fewer calories, being more physically active, or, best of all, a combination of the two."** [Emphasis added] *Dietary Guidelines for Americans 2010* at page 21.

The above sounds reasonable but is wrong. Gary Taubes, the *New York Times* award-winning journalist previously mentioned, wrote a seminal critique of the calories-in minus calories-out equation in *Good Calories, Bad Calories* (2007). He then summarized and continued his critique in his follow-on bestseller *Why We Get Fat, And What We Can Do About It* (2011). He bluntly stated at page 7 of *Why We Get Fat,* "Over the years, this calories-in/calories-out paradigm of excess fat has proved to be remarkably resistant to any evidence to the contrary." He went on " I will argue in this book that the fault lies entirely with the medical orthodoxy — both the belief that excess fat is caused by consuming excess calories, and the advice that stems from it." He lays out his critique with the following: "I'm going to argue that this calories-in/calories-out paradigm of adiposity [fat accumulation] is nonsensical, that **we don't get fat because we eat too much and move too little, and that we can't solve the problem by doing the opposite**." [Emphasis added] *Id.* at page 8. What does Taubes recommend to help us trim down and/or stay trim?

His conclusion: "The most fattening foods are the ones that have the greatest effect on our blood sugar and insulin levels. These are the concentrated sources of carbohydrates, and particularly those that we can digest quickly: anything made of refined flour (bread, cereals, and pasta), liquid carbohydrates (beers, fruit juices, and sodas), and starches (potatoes, rice, and corn)." *Id.* at pg.134. Why? "These foods flood the bloodstream quickly with glucose. Blood sugar shoots up: insulin shoots up. [The natural controls are overwhelmed.] We get fatter." *Id.* How long has this been generally known? "Not surprisingly, these foods have been considered uniquely fattening for nearly two hundred years...." *Id.* at pages 134-5.

That is pretty much all the diet advice you need to know to begin moving in the right direction. The key is to avoid the fattening foods identified by Gary Taubes and increase the amount of real whole food you consume. Of course there is more to it than having this simple knowledge in mind. The solution is fairly straightforward in concept, but easier said than done in practice, as we all know. It requires changes in daily behavior and change to established habit patterns is never easy.

More recently, author Jonathan Bailor extended the critique against "eat less and exercise more" as the answer to maintaining a healthy weight in *The Calorie Myth* (2014). Mr Bailor spent a decade reviewing the nutrition and exercise research contained in over 1200 worldwide studies and laid out his findings in *The Calorie Myth.* The book is a very succinct but counter-intuitive explanation of why the advice to "eat less and exercise more" does not work. His conclusions are based on the scientific literature not his personal hunches, anecdotal evidence or fragmented observations. Much of his evidence comes from well-controlled studies carried out by mainstream researchers. Bailor goes on to explain what does and does not work as documented in the scientific literature.

His advice is that calorie counting i.e. calorie restriction, as it is more properly labeled does not work over the long-term. This is not because we lack willpower but because the body will defend itself against calorie restriction by increasing hunger, slowing down the metabolism and slowing down physical activity. As an extra bonus you feel crummy. When the calorie counting ends, usually because of constant nagging hunger, the body will rebuild its fat stores very rapidly. That is why this strategy more often than not leads to net weight gain. Oops!

What works is increasing the real whole food in the diet and cutting out the processed and starchy foods just as Gary Taubes and others have concluded. In Bailor's formulation this leads to changing our "set point" so our bodies will use the fuel we provide from food more efficiently and not store fat. His specific nutrition recommendations are a bit more prescriptive than, but generally consistent with, a Paleo or Primal approach. He urges us to eat only "SANE" foods and skip the rest. Sane foods are those real whole foods that fill you up and provide all the proper nutrition you need. Whether his approach is right for you is a personal decision that you can make after reading his book. (Note- I found *The Calorie Myth* at my local library. Local libraries will usually order a book for you if it is not on hand already.) The value of *The Calorie Myth* is its synthesis and succinct presentation of so much documented scientific research and the simple nutrition advice Bailor derived from his decade of work. His conclusions are a direct challenge to the conventional wisdom most of us have learned over the years.

Bailor also makes recommendations on how to get the most from exercise. He recommends shorter more intense workouts to build healthy muscles as a component of overall health and wellness. Bailor debunks the notion that we need to spend hours every day in the gym in order to stay healthy. He recommends twenty-minute strength and interval workouts to build muscle. He explains the science behind how properly conditioned muscle tissue helps keep us healthy at the hormonal and cellular level above and beyond the aesthetics involved in a toned body. Again, whether his exercise recommendations will work for you is a personal decision but I commend his book for your thoughtful consideration.

Chapter Six- Why our evolutionary past matters.

"A lot of people try to think up ideas. I'm not one. I'd rather accept the irresistible possibilities of what I can't ignore." (Robert Rauschenberg, Artist)

Does the past matter? If so, how can knowledge of the past help us today? Jonathan Bailor illustrates why our evolutionary past matters in this brilliant passage from *The Calorie Myth*:

> "One way to clear up all the calorie confusion is to start at the beginning and look at the history of eating using a scale of one day. Say 12:00 a.m. [midnight] was the dawn of our first ancestors and right now it's one second before midnight. Up until 11:57 p.m. our ancestors stayed healthy and fit, eating only what could be found in nature— vegetables, seafood, meat, eggs, fruits, nuts and seeds. At 11:57 p.m. people started farming, became "civilized" and began eating starch and a small amount of sweets. Two seconds ago, people started eating processed starches and sweets. Only right now—one second before midnight— did people start getting most of their calories from genetically modified and highly manufactured starch — and sweetener based edible products." *The Calorie Myth* at page 94.

As Bailor cleverly shows, the past is not really past!

It is well established by genetic researchers that the past is alive today in our genes. While our genetic make-up is virtually identical to our pre-civilization ancestors from 10,000 years ago, we are living in a radically new food environment. The crux of the problem is that we have not had time to adapt genetically to this new food environment and may never adapt in a healthy way to this new environment. This situation was brought to light in an article almost 30 years ago in the prestigious New England Journal of Medicine titled *Paleolithic Nutrition: A Consideration of Its Nature and Current Implications* by S. Boyd Eaton, MD and Melvin Konner, PhD (1985). The doctors postulated, "... human beings today are confronted with diet-related health problems that were previously of minor importance and for which prior genetic adaptation has poorly prepared us." *New England Journal of Medicine* Vol. 312, No. 5, pg. 283. They went on to state "The human genetic constitution has changed relatively little since the appearance of truly modern human beings, *Homo Sapiens*, about 40,000 years ago." *Id.* Dr. Loren Cordain summed up the situation in *The Paleo Diet* by saying that we are Stone Age people living in the Space Age. Cordain pays tribute to the groundbreaking work of Eaton and Konner in inspiring his life-long academic research into Paleolithic nutrition. Geneticists using modern techniques have proven conclusively that our genetic make-up is virtually unchanged from our healthy Stone Age ancestors, validating Eaton's and Konner's early insights.

Study of the archeological record supports that our ancient ancestors were healthy and fit and could survive into their seventies or eighties if they did not succumb to accidents or other deadly misfortunes before that. The working hypothesis that flows from these observations is that we should take a serious look at our ancient ancestors daily nutrition (and other aspects of how they lived their lives) and consider using this information as a guide to what we should be eating now and otherwise doing for optimal health.

Chapter Seven- Debunking the myths about calories and nutrition.

As discussed earlier, Jonathan Bailor spent a decade studying over 1200 scientific studies in the worldwide literature on nutrition, exercise and health and presented his conclusions in the 2014 book *The Calorie Myth*. This book is an invaluable summary of and addition to our understanding of what the best scientific evidence is telling us right now about what to eat and how to exercise to attain wellness. By "wellness" I mean optimal health for a person factoring in their age and general physical condition. Clearly, we go through many physical changes as we go through life. Some are very significant such as the growth that occurs during childhood, the changes during puberty, changes during pregnancy and child bearing, and the more subtle changes that occur through the aging process during the latter stages of life. We know our health and physical condition are never constant. We may also suffer injuries or illnesses that disable us over the short- or long-term. Nevertheless, we can take common sense steps to optimize our health and wellness at any time even as our overall physical condition changes over time.

According to Bailor several persistent belief systems (myths) tend to drive current nutrition advice and our thinking. They are the following: (1) Weight loss = Calories in minus Calories out; (2) A Calorie is a Calorie; (3) All Foods Are Fine in Moderation; and (4) Exercising More Will Make You Thin. Bailor demolishes all of these myths using the best nutrition and exercise research available today.

The most persistent myth is that calorie counting, i.e. calorie restriction will lead to weight loss. The science does not support this conclusion and our own real life experience probably doesn't either. The problem with this myth is basic. The belief that our bodies operate like a thermodynamic machine is not supported by reality. According to Bailor, when we restrict calories three things tend to happen. First, we get hungry. Second, we get tired as the body seeks to suppress physical activity. And, third, our overall metabolism slows down so we burn fewer calories. And we probably get more than a little bit cranky. Bailor calls this natural response to a calorie restricting diet, increasing your "set point" weight. This increase is the opposite of the desired result. These same things happen with laboratory animals whose calorie intake is reduced in perfectly controlled environments. The net result is some early weight loss that tends to taper off followed by rapid weight gain once the unnatural and unsustainable state of calorie restriction and persistent hunger ends. Yo-yo dieting does not work and we all know it. More perplexing is why people continue to put their hopes in this strategy.

The second and third myths are closely related and, as Bailor demonstrates, do not square with the scientifically valid research. The idea that a "calorie is a calorie" is inconsistent with the growing body of knowledge about how different foods are digested, metabolized and eventually put to work by our bodies. This persistent myth also defies common sense. Bailor shows how different foods affect our hormones, primarily the master hormone insulin, and how different types of food are either good sources of nutrition and health promotion or the opposite. He uses the acronym "SANE" to differentiate healthy "sane" foods from unhealthy "insane" foods. Fat storage, the result we want to avoid, is one of the results of eating what Bailor calls "insane" foods. Clearly, if some foods are "sane" and some are "insane" because of the health promoting quality or health destroying effect they cause, it follows directly that some foods in any amount are not good for us.

The third myth that "all foods are fine in moderation" is also refuted by the above simple logic about how different foods affect our bodies. Some products marketed as food are harmful in any amount. "Trans fats" are one example. Once ubiquitous in the American diet they have been largely removed from products as the evidence piled up against the product. However they are still incorporated in some processed foods. In addition, we tend to be quite adept at redefining "moderation" to suit our own desires and needs resulting in immoderate "moderation" especially when it comes to snacks and other tasty "insane" foods. Donuts anyone?

Bailor lays out his recommendations on the "sane" foods we should consume and in what proportions. He recommends that nonstarchy vegetables should form the base of your "sane" food pyramid, followed by nutrient-dense proteins, whole-food fats and low-fructose fruits. *The Calorie Myth* page 132. As far as the foods to avoid, he indicts the same suspects as other informed sources. These are the foods that produce elevated blood sugar spikes and result in fat buildup — primarily refined sugar and refined grain products.

The forth myth is often closely linked with the first. As I recounted in my journey back to health in Chapter One my doctor's advice to "eat better and get more exercise" is the conventional wisdom that is reflected in most of the weight-loss solutions promoted in the marketplace and by most healthcare professionals. By "more exercise" this usually means burning more calories through aerobic exercise. We are told to increase the time spent on the exercise bike, jogging or on the elliptical burning up more calories — the more the better. As all gym goers know, modern exercise equipment conveniently has a "calories burned" readout that is the last thing to check when the workout is over. Unfortunately, these readouts are estimates with little practical value. But there is a bigger problem with this approach.

Bailor questions the idea that we just need to put in more hours doing intensive aerobic workouts. He points out that the body's response to increased aerobic exercise is similar to when we restrict calories to lose weight. Our body is too smart for this approach and sees the increased exercise load as a challenge to the status quo. Our body reacts by increasing hunger as we "work up our appetites." This leads to higher calorie consumption than would otherwise occur. *The Calorie Myth* Chapter 5. The net result is no weight loss. Also, loads and loads of cardio work is physically draining. Bailor does not leave you high and dry however. He has detailed advice on how to work out smarter to build hormonally sound muscle tissue that actually aids in long-term weight control and health promotion. *The Calorie Myth* chapters 21-2. Again, I recommend his book and its exercise model for your consideration.

Chapter Eight- Food consumption in the United States — the real food pyramid is a real problem.

Let's take a look at what the typical American diet generally includes, according to the federal government's USDA economic research service.

"USDA's Economic Research Service (ERS) estimates that [the] dietary intake of calories in 2000 [was] just under 2,700 calories per person per day. ERS data suggest that average daily calorie intake increased by 24.5 percent, or about 530 calories, between 1970 and 2000. Of that 24.5-percent increase, grains (mainly refined grain products) contributed 9.5 percentage points [39% of the increase]; added fats and oils, 9.0 percentage points [37% of the increase]; added sugars, 4.7 percentage points [19% of the increase]; fruits and vegetables together, 1.5 percentage points; meats and nuts together, 1 percentage point; and dairy products and eggs together, 1.5 percentage point."

In other words, the bulk of the increase in calories has come from refined grains, added fats and oils and added sugar [95% of the increase]. As discussed earlier, calories do matter but not all calories are created equal. The facts show that the worst calories from a weight loss/maintenance perspective are those that are increasing in consumption the most in the US.

As discussed earlier, some experts believe that **sugar consumption is <u>the</u> <u>problem</u>** driving increases in obesity and obesity's associated chronic diseases. Other knowledgeable sources believe refined grains are the main problem. These two conclusions are not contradictory. Both sugar and refined grains are a big part of the problem. The only debate is over which is the bigger problem.

The USDA report went on: "Now more than ever, America is a Nation of meat eaters. In 2000, total meat consumption (red meat, poultry, and fish) reached 195 pounds (boneless, trimmed- weight equivalent) per person, 57 pounds above average annual consumption in the 1950s." The report attributed this increase mainly to growing prosperity.

And: "In 2000, Americans drank an average of 38 percent less milk and ate nearly four times as much cheese (excluding cottage, pot, and baker's cheese) as in the 1950s." The report attributed the reduction in milk drinking to "Consumption of soft drinks, fruit drinks and ales, and flavored teas may be displacing beverage milk in the diet. Big increases in eating away from home, especially at fast-food places, and in consumption of salty snack foods favored soft drink consumption." Plus, "Lifestyles that emphasize convenience foods were probably major forces behind the higher consumption [of cheese]. In fact, more than half of our cheese now comes in commercially manufactured and prepared foods (including food service), such as pizza, tacos, nachos, salad bars, fast- food sandwiches, bagel spreads, sauces for baked potatoes and other vegetables, and packaged snack foods. Advertising and new products—such as reduced-fat cheeses and resealable bags of shredded cheeses, including cheese blends tailored for use in Italian and Mexican recipes— also boosted consumption."

One more finding regarding oils: "Americans in 2000 consumed, on average, three-and-three-fifths times more salad and cooking oil than they did annually in the 1950s, and more than twice as much shortening." Why? "By 1999, the fats and oils group's contribution to total fat had jumped 12 percentage points to 53 percent, probably due to the higher consumption of fried foods in foodservice outlets, the increase in consumption of high-fat snack foods, and the increased use of salad dressings. Margarine, salad dressings and mayonnaise, cakes and other sweet baked goods, and oils continue to appear in the top 10 foods for fat contribution, according to recent USDA food intake surveys, which indicates the ongoing prevalence of discretionary fats in Americans' diets." Whoa, hold on there my friend, I'm not sure I want fries with that!

It should not be a surprise that this data is in line with the government's recommendations to eat more grains and in line with the predicted causal effect of sugar subsidies and with the changes the food industry has made to adapt to this evolving environment.

This report demonstrates that the federal government is a key player in shaping food production and consumption in the US. Obviously, the food industry is acutely aware of the government's role. In fact, the food industry is constantly adjusting its output to respond to consumer tastes (many of which the industry is driving) and government policy. More on this later. There would be nothing inherently wrong with this situation if the beneficial results were proving out in our health trends as expected from the government's recommendations. But we know that this is not the case.

A June 2015 article in Time magazine chronicled that, on average, adult Americans now weigh 30 pounds more that adult Americans did in 1960. Again, the question is why this is happening and what can be done to correct this unfortunate trend?

As I developed earlier, the excessive consumption of refined grains and refined sugar, including HFCS, are the main suspects in the escalating obesity crisis in our country. Even if the case were not conclusive against refined grains and sugar at this point, it would be prudent for government planners to redirect research dollars toward a fair examination of the question of why our population-based health is not improving and toward a fair examination of any alternative hypotheses that might help explain what is going on. As Gary Taubes explained in *Good Calories, Bad Calories*, our government and the research funding it controls continue to be directed toward a stubborn hypothesis that dietary fat is driving increased cholesterol and resultant heart disease. This theory has not proven out after many years of directed research and billions of dollars spent.

As we all understand at some level, the United States has a complex web of interrelationships between food producers, food processors, food distributors and the restaurant industry, collectively the "food industry," and the government. These interrelationships exist within a regulatory framework administered by the federal Food and Drug Administration (FDA) and other federal and state government agencies and, as previously discussed, are impacted by federal nutrition policy from the DHHS and USDA. The food industry works closely with its advocates (lobbyists and lawyers) and trade associations (organized lobbying structures) to make sure the federal agencies do not take any action that will damage their financial interests. This makes perfect sense for them. But is this good for the average consumer? Do consumers have a voice in this complex mix? If so, how effectively is the consumer's voice represented in established government policy? Are there ways average citizens can make their voices more heard in this complex environment? I will have some thoughts on this in later chapters.

Chapter Nine- How to get healthier starting today.

What concepts have we covered so far?

Most important is that there is a growing body of scientifically valid international research that points us in the right direction to reclaim our health and wellness at any age. The nutrition concepts are actually fairly straightforward. They have been well known folk wisdom for many years. The problem is these potential solutions were lost amongst a deluge of conflicting information over the last few generations and especially since the federal government weighed-in on the topic with the McGovern Committee Report in 1977 and subsequent nutrition recommendations.

My research and personal experience over the past months convinced me to travel back to the future and build my nutrition around the real whole foods that sustained our ancient ancestors before we became "civilized" and overly dependent on the processed foods our current food industry produces and promotes.

As discussed earlier, I am a huge fan of the approach advanced by Mark Sisson in *The Primal Blueprint*. His approach is sensible and based on good science. It advances a commonsensical program that is flexible. Primal nutrition does not demand that you never eat another potato chip the rest of your life. Just don't eat too many of them or too often. *The Primal Blueprint* provides a practical solution that has the promise to deliver long-term sustainable health and wellness.

We have learned that the conventional wisdom to "eat better and get more exercise" is incomplete, at best, and possibly leading us in the wrong direction. We now know that calorie restriction absolutely does not work over the long-term. Long sessions on the treadmill or other exercise equipment to burn calories tend to wear us down and generally do not trim weight long-term. So what does work?

What works is to eat real whole food and exercise smarter. My research and personal experience leads to this simple nutrition advice— **eat more real whole food and skip the processed stuff**. This advice includes a recommendation to drastically reduce, if not eliminate, refined grains; and to drastically reduce refined sugar intake. On the exercise front— add some shorter more intense strength and interval training with needed rest in between so the body can recover fully and you are on your way to significantly better health and wellness. More daily movement and more walking are important to health, as are healthy relationships at work and at home. Add some stress reducing activities and a good night's sleep as often as possible and you are on your way. Wow, who knew?

These are the ideas that come from taking an *Evolution Health* perspective to nutrition and exercise. My personal recommendations are contained in Appendix A and are offered for your consideration.

Chapter Ten- Sorting through the best diet advice on the market— a guidebook to low carbohydrate diets.

A great place to start your search for a solid low carbohydrate diet that suits your personality is *Living Low Carb* by Jonney Bowden, PhD, CNS (2013). The book reviews the top 23 low carbohydrate diets and explains how they might work, or not work, for different personality types. This simplifies the job of randomly choosing a diet/lifestyle plan that might work for you from among the thousands out in the commercial marketplace (most of which will probably not help you achieve your long term goals).

Living Low Carb guides you through the better-known low carb approaches. I am proceeding on the premise that the previous chapters have convinced you that low carb diets work. Or at least on the premise that a suitable low carb diet deserves an honest try to see if it will work for you. The low carb genre includes many popular diets — Atkins, Dukan, South Beach, Paleo, Primal, The Zone and others. Each has a slightly different approach and some have been around many years. This is not a one size fits all world so its best to make a choice that holds out the promise of success for you. Your hairdresser or barber may need a different solution.

What is success? I assume that first goal on most people's list is weight loss. Second, I would suggest feeling better and being objectively healthier, i.e. wellness. Third is sustainability. Almost any diet can deliver some weight loss in a certain period of time. But what if you feel worse, are always fatigued and constantly hungry? Game over and back to the old patterns. And usually a net weight gain comes along as an added bonus. This approach does not bring sustainable wellness. Finally I assume, none of us is looking to join a religious order that demands rigid allegiance to a difficult lifestyle. That's a different book!

Flexibility is very important to me and will be for many of you. Simplicity is a must. As I described earlier, my choice came down to *The Primal Blueprint* by Mark Sisson. In my view it is by far the best Paleo inspired book on the market, especially for those over 50 (the author recently turned 60). The book is clearly written with summaries at the beginning and end of each chapter. It has great graphics to illustrate the main points. It provides an innovative approach to exercise that is easy and provides effective workout suggestions. The exercise recommendations involve more intense strength and interval training that can be completed in about 20 minutes per session a few times per week — no more endless cardio workouts. This exercise approach is very similar to that recommended by Jonathan Bailor in *The Calorie Myth*. Both authors stress that proper exercise will increase the muscles' built-in capacity to regulate hormones and control/reduce fat accumulation that results from hormonal imbalances driven by bad nutrition. Mark Sisson also has a very robust website Marksdailyapple.com that has many supporting posts to help you maintain your enthusiasm on the journey that will involve ups and downs. The free website includes helpful videos that demonstrate his exercise suggestions. I find that seeing the exercises in video format is far superior to reading about them in a book and hoping I am getting it right.

So I recommend that you take a look at Jonny Bowdin's excellent survey, *Living Low Carb,* and decide which of the 23 most popular low carb diets might work for you. Then put your choice to the test. If *The Primal Blueprint* holds out promise for you, go for it.

Part Three- Building your personal toolkit to improve your health and wellness.

Chapter Eleven- Reviewing the basic building blocks.

In earlier chapters I reviewed the relevant literature that has informed my personal approach to nutrition and exercise. I highlighted those authors and researchers who, I believe, are providing the best advice today. I also related my personal experience with a Paleo/Primal approach in Chapter One and why I think it is worth your time to understand this approach and consider applying it in your daily routine.

It is a daunting task to sort through all the nutrition and exercise advice on the market. Go into any large bookstore and you'll see entire sections devoted to diet and exercise. Each book is claiming the mantle and seeks to move you toward spending your hard earned money on the advice. We know that many of these books are passing fads, soon forgotten with next month's shipment.

Some key questions are. Will the advice produce the desired results? Can I actually do it given my current lifestyle and the other demands on my time and resources? Does it mesh with my culture, background and lifestyle? Is it truly health promoting or just a quick fix? Can I stick with it over the long-term and lock-in the benefits? Will I feel empowered or deprived? Will I feel healthier?

That is a long list of criteria and each point is important to consider. My bias brings me back to the question of how persuasive is the body of research supporting the approach? Is it based on one person's observations or many data points over a large data set, possibly including numerous clinically valid controlled studies? Many of the diet books fail right out of the gate to meet this important threshold because they rely on a small sample size and then extrapolate that limited experience across the entire American consumer base.

As previously discussed, *The Paleo Diet* and *The Calorie Myth* are two of the best sources of scientifically valid research on nutrition and exercise on the market. Together these books summarize and provide access to regular people (non-scientists) about what the state of the art nutritional science has discovered. And while these two books conclude with slightly different approaches to nutrition and exercise they are consistent in providing the basic building blocks to better health.

What are the building blocks? First is to eat real whole food and skip the processed stuff. Second is to tone the large muscles in the body with more intense but shorter strength training. Third is to do some short intense interval training from time to time to build cardiovascular health. Fourth is to move more every day as we go about our daily routines. Maximize walking about. Fifth is to add some stress reducing activities to our weekly habits. My personal favorite is Yoga, which I will discuss more later. Next, maintain healthy relationships at home and at work. Finally, get a good night's sleep as often as possible. These simple steps will work if they become a part of our routines. Each will be explored more in-depth in the chapters that follow.

The Paleo/Primal idea is based on sound science developed over many years and is consistent with the logic of evolution. The conclusion that we are not genetically adapted to thrive on processed food is clearly established to my satisfaction. Our bodies need real whole food. There is an increasing body of valid research adding depth to our understanding about how our modern food supply is probably the cause of many of the common chronic diseases that negatively affect Americans.

One major problem in consuming processed food is we don't even know what is contained in many processed food products so it is impossible to make good judgments about them. *Eat It to Beat It* by David Zinczenko (2013) points out "... there are more than 3,000 food additives approved by the FDA...." *Eat It to Beat It* at page 6.

But he goes on to describe that the federal government's approval process contains a very large loophole that allows food manufactures to declare that an additive is "generally recognized as safe [GRAS]" and bring the additive to market with minimal oversight. *Id.* I took a course in FDA law in my graduate law program and found the regulatory scheme out of date and confusing. Many informed observers believe it is inadequate to protect consumers from potentially harmful food additives. And, my studies in the mid nineteen eighties were well before the GMO issue came into focus.

In addition to a weak regulatory scheme and the problems with food labels, we are confronted with a dizzying list of ingredients in many processed foods that would challenge a PhD in chemistry to understand, let alone the average consumer. Another question arises: each food additive is a chemical or organic substance by itself that may or may not have been adequately tested for safety before it was used, but what about any potential negative interactions among the many additives?

Another big problem is that government regulations and guidelines allow labeling that is confusing at best and downright fraudulent at worst. For example, food can be labeled "zero trans fats" as long as the trans fats do not exceed a certain threshold amount. I don't know about you but "zero" should mean zero. [Note: the federal government recently issued regulations intended to remove trans fats from the food supply but this change will be phased in over a number of years, if the regulations stand up over time.]

Another example of the shortcomings of food labels is illustrated by the "gluten free" craze. In some cases, the gluten is removed and replaced by substances that are as bad as gluten or worse. And "gluten free" is used to tout unhealthy products that never contained gluten in the first place, such as potato chips fried in low quality vegetable oils. We all know that the "low fat" and "low/no cholesterol" foods of prior decades did not produce better health trends across the US population. These products were aggressively marketed as being healthier than the alternatives and were fully consistent with the federal government's guidelines. The reality was (and still is) these products were not always healthy. The same scenario is playing out with the newer approved marketing labels and there will likely be more of the same in the future. Caution and healthy skepticism is in order when interpreting popular food labels.

So what is the best advice? My conclusion is to generally avoid the challenges of label reading and go with real whole food. While label reading has value, it is not foolproof. Keep it simple. Real whole food does not need a label to explain it. Broccoli is broccoli. Celery is celery. An apple is an apple. Fresh salmon is fresh salmon. Butter is butter. Real whole food is the food our hunter-gatherer ancestors would easily recognize, not to mention the food our grandparents would recognize. Once you leave this safe and nutritious zone and venture into the processed food wonderland it is hard to know what you are eating.

Chapter Twelve- Being more intentional about the food we buy, prepare and consume.

"Whether you like it or not, everything that is happening to you at this moment is a result of the choices you've made in the past. Unfortunately, a lot of us make choices unconsciously, and therefore we don't think they are choices — and yet, they are." Deepak Chopra MD, *The Seven Spiritual Laws of Success* at page 40.

Dr. Chopra may not be your favorite personal guru but his insight is valuable. Every time we chose to go in one direction we chose not to go in the many alternative directions available at that moment. A key to making good choices is our intention before we make the choice. What are we trying to achieve with the choice? What alternatives exist? What is the best choice? Do I have enough information? How do I decide? Do I have to make tradeoffs due to budgetary constraints?

Much of the food purchasing in our country is the result of marketing and conditioning that result in unconscious decision-making. Dr. Choopra says, "Most of us, as result of conditioning, have repetitious and predictable responses to the stimuli in our environment." *The Seven Spiritual Laws of Success* at page 41. "We are simply making these choices unconsciously." *Id.* We frequently make our grocery shopping decisions on impulse or habit without much thought, pulling the same products off the shelves that we are used to buying. That unconscious decision-making process can and frequently does lead to a shopping cart loaded with substandard foods.

Intentional grocery shopping is one of the most powerful tools we can bring to the effort to reclaim and protect our health. As I recounted in Chapter One, I had been cruising along on autopilot accepting the conventional wisdom about nutrition and health. This wisdom taught that a "balanced diet" where you did not consume too many calories and where you included plenty of whole grains would bring the best results. This conventional wisdom also included the implicit idea that a slow decline toward chronic disease was inevitable unless you were one of the lucky few that had magical protection in their genes or from some other mysterious source beyond our influence. The result was that, like many people, I went along with the flow and hoped to slow down the inevitable decline but had to learn to accept a less than robust future.

My autopilot food purchasing was a big part of the problem. I bought food products based on promotions, product placement and habit — external stimuli. When I became dissatisfied with this worldview, as described earlier, I set out to see if there was a healthier way. As I reported, I found one, put it to work for me and got the positive results I was seeking. A basic component of this better way was smarter, more intentional grocery shopping.

I decided to be more intentional about the food I purchased, brought into my home, prepared and consumed. I had to break some old habits. I no longer buy the 2 for 1 "specials" on snacks, bread and other goodies. Actually, I rarely go down the interior aisles of the grocery store these days or wander around the bakery section because I don't want to trigger those old cravings and fall back into unhealthy habit patterns.

So step one is to harness your positive willpower. Set your intention and make the commitment to buying healthy food and foregoing the unhealthy items before you go to market. As I have repeated many times for emphasis, the goal is to maximize the real whole food and skip the processed stuff. The step before this is to plan ahead before you head out to the grocery store or farmer's market. Prepare a weekly meal plan and shop to carry out the plan. There are plenty of cookbooks available to help you make quick and easy healthy meals. I have listed some suggestions in Appendix B. Make sure you have what you will need in your pantry and kitchen to efficiently prepare tasty food during the week. Instead of impulse buying at the grocery store based on product placement and pricing specials have a list that will cover more than a few days' meals and then stick with it. An added benefit to this approach is probably lower food bills overall.

Next is to enjoy food preparation and consumption. Make food preparation a regular part of your weekly and daily routines. Get the whole family involved. Especially if you have children, use the opportunity to spend time together. Chop, peal, smash, count, measure and otherwise have fun in the kitchen. Sing songs, whistle while you work and play games. Turn a chore into an opportunity to strengthen your family ties.

My wife and I were told when our son was in kindergarten that one of the few reliable predictors of academic success for children was whether the children had dinner together with their parents on a regular basis. I believe that preparing the evening meal together and eating mindfully together brings a host of benefits beyond just good nutrition. It adds to your quality of life. It's fun. Best of all it does not cost anything extra and will most likely save you money.

The cover story in the October 20, 2014 *Time Magazine* was titled "The Truth about Home Cooking- A Guide to Taking Back Your Kitchen" by best selling author and current *New York Times* food writer Mark Bittman. He cites some numbers about the poor state of nutrition in the US and states "Cooking real food is the best defense — not to mention that any meal you're likely to eat at home contains about 200 fewer calories than one you would eat at a restaurant. " October 20, 2014 *Time Magazine* at page 52. He also has a different take on the profusion of food shows: "Making food a performance, as entertaining as that can be from our seats in the grandstand, has had a damaging effect on our relationship to cooking." *Id.* His answer — do some preplanning and do it yourself, together with your family or a small group. As the subtitle to his article says, we need to "take back" our kitchens. I couldn't agree more. Keep your food sources real and have fun re-inhabiting the real estate you are already paying for.

None of the above will happen without setting your specific intention. By being thoughtful about planning ahead for grocery shopping; about the food you buy and bring into your home; and setting aside special time to prepare and share meals together, as often as possible, you will strengthen your family bonds. Who knows, maybe your children will even do better in school. At the very least, they will learn to be contributing members of your family and that will bring everyone more peace of mind and joy.

Chapter Thirteen- Cost/benefit considerations in purchasing nutritious whole food.

It is difficult, if not impossible, to make apples to apples comparisons between real whole food and processed food. The challenge here is similar to testing one nutrition hypothesis against another in an uncontrolled environment.

What follows is not an economist's study of the cost comparison issue but rather some food for thought in making purchasing decisions. The recent *Time Magazine* article I quoted above stated "And to save money and still eat well you don't need local, organic ingredients, all you need is real food. I'm not saying local food isn't better, it is. But there is plenty of decent food in the more than 37,000 grocery stores in the US." October 20, 2014 *Time Magazine* at page 53.

It is obvious that on an item-by-item basis real whole food is often more expensive than the mass-produced, highly processed variety. For example, high quality artisanal cheese is a lot more expensive than the grocery store brand. We know that certified organic products are more expensive than non-organic. But these obvious examples do not answer the question of whether real, nutritious, whole food is worth it when all the costs are considered and when cost mitigating strategies are pursued. An economist doing a real and complete comparison would have to consider the fully loaded costs versus the price at the checkout counter to come to valid conclusions. What should be factored into the equation beyond the price you pay?

First is the intangible but very important factor— quality. What goes into making a judgment about quality? There are many factors but taste, texture, how the food makes you feel one, two or three hours later, and enjoyment of the food when it is consumed enter into the analysis. Is it from nature or loaded with additives? Quality is highly subjective and highly personal but we know it is important even if it cannot be quantified down to the penny. Why are wine connoisseurs willing to pay many hundreds or even thousands of dollars more for a special bottle of wine? Beyond the possible snob appeal, the wine must deliver a higher quality experience or it will not command a premium price for very long— that is how quality plays out in real world comparisons. We know it when we experience it and when we don't.

A second factor in comparing costs is the need to include any derivative costs that can be traced directly to the food we consume. A major point of this book and the Primal/Paleo movement is that we can regain our health by feeding our bodies the wholesome food it needs to maintain optimal health. This will increase our odds against developing chronic diseases such as diabetes, heart disease, neurological disease and some cancers. Many disabling but preventable chronic diseases are caused by poor lifestyle choices, especially including poor nutrition. Our government acknowledges this fact. If the costs of these preventable conditions is factored into our food purchasing costs the slightly higher sticker price of healthier choices minus the cost of chronic diseases would win the cost comparison every time. However, the potential costs of chronic disease are deferred. The costs of treating chronic disease will occur later, even much later if at all, so it is easy to disregard these costs while we grocery shop. But I believe these costs are just as real as the amount we pay at checkout and should be considered in evaluating your grocery budget and your long-term budget strategy for medical treatment.

Plus there are purchasing strategies that can lower the cost of real whole food. Buying in bulk. Food exchanges and co-ops are making progress on this front. These approaches have the added benefit of bringing communities together. And of course the Internet has a growing number of sources of real whole food at prices below what you might pay at the grocery store. The new company Thrive Market® is an example.

Finally, you may have heard that one of the leading American whole food purveyors, not coincidentally, named Whole Foods Market® has made the strong case that shopping with them is not more expensive than the national chains, if you shop smart.

Their website has a tab called "The Whole Deal®" devoted to helping customers shop at their stores and do it on a budget.

Interestingly, Whole Foods Market® recently opened a large store in Detroit, a community not known as affluent. I'm not picking on Detroit, but the city has well documented economic problems. The point is that the savvy grocer Whole Foods Market® has made a real world bet that the residents of Detroit will be able to afford and will patronize what many consider an upscale grocer. Whole Foods has run the numbers to be sure and would not have opened this store in Detroit if things did not add up. I wish them success and better health for their new customers.

Chapter Fourteen- The role of reasonable, regular exercise and restful sleep.

Regular exercise is on everyone's list of activities to build a healthier body, especially right after New Year's Day. The practical questions are: what kind of exercise will do the most good with the shortest investment of time?

Most people don't have the luxury of spending hours at the gym every day. Most people do not want to spend hours every day working-out even if they theoretically have the time. So what works best?

My research led me to some surprising results about the most effective exercise program to practice to maintain optimal health. First, as Jonathan Bailor explained in *The Calorie Myth* increasing aerobic exercise as a way to control or lose weight generally does not work because our bodies have natural defenses against this strategy that tend to win the struggle over the long run. The scientific evidence he discusses leads to the conclusion that we tend to eat more calories to compensate for the increased energy expenditures. Our bodies sense the increased energy demand and this stimulates hunger. Increased hunger leads to more calorie intake than would otherwise occur. Net result — weight stabilization or gain.

Bailor is a strong proponent of regular exercise but of a markedly different type than most mainstream exercise professionals recommend. His exercise recommendations include regular intense strength training and some regular intense interval training. His workouts take about 20 minutes each including warm-up and cool down periods. He explores the concept of eccentric exercise versus concentric exercise. In brief, eccentric exercise moves the large muscles slowly through expanding motions. Concentric exercise is the opposite where the large muscles contract, as during arm curls with barbells. He provides the science behind his view that eccentric exercises build all of the four types of muscle fibers whereas concentric exercises only work one of the four types of muscle fiber, the fast twitch fibers. By working all of the muscle fibers simultaneously we get better results at the cellular and hormonal levels. This helps put our bodies in balance and strengthens our complex hormone system as a defense against fat accumulation.

In a New Year's Eve story December 31, 2014 in the New York Times online titled *The Super-Short Workout and Other Fitness Trends* the author catalogued a growing trend in the fitness world — much shorter but more intense workout programs. The science behind this trend is considerable and growing.

Mark Sisson advocates a similar workout pattern in *The Primal Blueprint*. He recommends regular intense strength training using more traditional exercise patterns. He calls his workout pattern the "lift heavy things" approach based on what our Paleo/Primal ancestors did each day to find food, prepare lodging and do other daily chores just to stay alive. He also recommends some regular intense interval training modeled after his observations of Olympic caliber sprinters he has seen in Southern California. This interval work is short full-out sprinting followed by recovery intervals and is similar to sprinting after or from animals back in the Paleo era. Both the strength work and the intervals can be completed in about 20 minutes from start to finish. My personal pattern is derived from Sisson's written descriptions in *The Primal Blueprint* and videos on Marksdailyapple.com with a dash of the eccentric movements inspired by Jonathan Bailor.

There are other benefits to regular exercise that may not be as well known. In the recently published book, *A Nation in Pain* (2014) Judy Foreman addresses the massive problem of chronic pain in our country. She cites numbers as high 100 million Americans who are living with chronic pain. This includes forty percent of all adults in our country. The major pain issues are: lower back pain, arthritis and fibromyalgia. In Chapter 13 she calls exercise "the real magic bullet" to alleviating chronic pain or at least helping people cope better with their conditions. She states plainly that "... the idea that exercise overall improves pain is settled science."

Again the question becomes: What kind of exercise helps most?" *A Nation in Pain* at page 288 provides the science. A review of "… 16 randomized controlled trials involving 1,730 people with chronic low back pain found that strength training is a particularly effective way to reduce pain" *Id.* Furthermore, her research revealed that supervised, fairly intense exercise for about 20 minutes was most effective in relieving back pain. This is consistent with Jonathan Bailor's and Mark Sisson's advice to increase intensity and decrease time spent in an exercise session.

A Nation in Pain discusses the benefits of exercise in dealing with pain from arthritis and fibromyalgia that parallel the results documented for lower back pain. *Id.* at pages 291-6.

Mark Sisson also recommends getting out to walk as often as possible. This is based on the observation that our Paleo/Primal ancestors did a lot of walking just about every day to find food and survive. They also did sprint work from time to time to escape danger or to hunt prey. And they lifted things and climbed obstacles naturally as part of their daily lives. All of these elements inform a Primal approach to regular exercise.

Another popular way to improve our health is Yoga. The ancient art of Yoga has many layers from the physical to the spiritual. As a form of exercise regular Yoga promises to increase flexibility, balance and body tone (muscle health). Yoga is a proven stress reliever and has the power to improve health and bring more emotional balance to our lives. Some Yoga approaches are specifically designed and advertised as "restorative." Other approaches are up-tempo and designed to provide an aerobic experience. And some newer approaches like "hot" Yoga are designed to bring up the body temperature and bring out the sweat. Because Yoga is very popular in the US today it is easy to find low cost options in most areas and find a style that suits you. Many gyms provide guided Yoga sessions as part of a reasonable monthly fee.

Yoga also has a deep spiritual element for those so inclined. In fact, Yoga can become an all-encompassing way of life if one chooses to immerse completely in its multi-layered richness. It's worth a look for those who have never tried it.

One of the most important reasons to get regular exercise is that it reduces stress and helps bring more balance to our otherwise hectic modern lives. Greater balance and less stress generally create a happier outlook and an increased ability to deal with life's inevitable challenges. We know the challenges will come, so improving our ability to handle them before they hit is a critical life skill that needs to be in everyone's toolkit.

In addition to regular exercise we need to focus on restful sleep. A good night's sleep as often as possible will augment the benefits of regular exercise. Our bodies need time to rebuild and rejuvenate. Restful sleep is a tonic we need to enjoy everyday.

Chapter Fifteen- Reducing stress through stronger personal relationships.

There is an impressive body of research about the negative effects of chronic stress on modern day Americans. Again, a look back into our evolutionary past is instructive. When danger threatened our ancient ancestors they naturally reacted with what we now call the "fight or flight" response. This hormonal response enabled them to deal with the threat by either confronting it or running away. Strong physiological processes were triggered that helped preserve our species from extinction. We still have this same built-in physiological response but the vast majority of triggers are no longer life threatening, at least not immediately. Stress can become chronic when the fight or flight response is triggered repeatedly every day. The negative effects of chronic stress build over time.

What are some of the most frequent stressors? Traffic jams, being late for meetings, work evaluations, work presentations, job interviews, turmoil at home or in the office, difficult deadlines, money worries, health concerns, the nightly news — the list is endless. We all have stressors. They come with our modern high-speed lives. The problem arises when these stressors are chronic, not just the occasional response to a life threatening event. So what are the strategies to achieve chronic stress reduction?

I spent some time talking about the stress busting value of regular exercise and Yoga above, but what about personal relationships? You may not have not heard about the "Roseto Effect." The name comes from a study of a group of men in the town of Roseto, Pennsylvania conducted in the 1960s. The study group consisted of the residents of this small town in Eastern Pennsylvania. The reason the group was interesting was because the residents were much less likely to die of heart disease than the American population in general. In fact, the men of Roseto between the ages of 55 and 64 were virtually immune to heart attacks. Men over the age of 65 had a mortality rate from heart attacks that was half the national average. See *The Great Cholesterol Myth* by Jonny Bowden PhD and Steven Sinatra, MD (2012) at page 150.

On closer scrutiny the reasons for these anomalies became clear. The men were mainly mineworkers who worked physically difficult jobs in nearby slate mines. Their nutrition was far from ideal and almost all the men were smokers. So how did men fitting this profile achieve drastically better mortality outcomes against heart attacks than average American men living throughout the country? The researchers made some key observations: most homes were multigenerational; families took strolls together most nights; the resident's had rich social connections with their neighbors through many existing clubs, churches and organized events; and even though the evening meal featured fried food and other "unhealthy" foods the dinner table provided a rich daily environment for personal interactions and nourishment of the human spirit. *Id.* at pages 150-60.

We can learn from the residents of Roseto. The essential take-away is that we need healthy personal relationships to sustain us. Relationships are not just nice to have; they are essential to human health. Our ancient ancestors understood this and their social arrangements naturally supported this basic human need. The challenge these days is finding the time to nurture the important relationships in our lives. Modern life pulls us in many directions. Keeping focus on healthy relationships with our fellow human beings (and pets too) is critical to staying healthy. It is one more way to break through chronic stress.

How are you doing in this area of your life?

Chapter Sixteen- Becoming better healthcare consumers through effective partnerships with our healthcare providers.

As I recounted in the introduction, I spent over 25 years in healthcare delivery, regulation and insurance first with the US Navy and later with some of the most recognizable firms in the country. I observed our healthcare system from several different perspectives that inform my outlook today.

The truth is I was a fairly standard healthcare consumer who used the system when I had problems and for occasional regular check-ups. I followed the typical model of waiting for advice from my doctors and other professionals about what I should do to stay healthy. I expected them to give me the information I needed without asking. Unfortunately, their input and advice was not always forthcoming or all that useful. Sometimes there was very little real advice at all. I don't follow or recommend a passive approach anymore.

As I recounted in Chapter One, the standard advice to "eat better and get more exercise" is more than a little vague and subject to interpretation. And most of us are very good at interpreting information and events in a way that reinforces our beliefs and habits rather than challenging them. Many healthcare professionals find it easier not to upset their patients with challenging recommendations. Most of us tend to operate on the assumption (hope) that there is or will be a magic pill or procedure to cure any problem that comes up and it will be available when we need it. I know I thought this way for most of my life. This worldview is the one I operated with for many years but no longer do because it does not work well as a strategy to prevent chronic disease.

Here is what I believe is a better model. We need to become smarter healthcare consumers (otherwise known as patients) by actively partnering with our healthcare professionals. Waiting patiently and submissively for the doctor to save us after chronic disease sets in is clearly not working for many Americans as earlier chapters demonstrated. And the economic costs of this treatment model are huge. The costs are growing alarmingly with no end in sight.

My new approach involved becoming more aware of the science behind how nutrition and exercise impacted my health. But awareness alone was not sufficient. Action was needed. I needed to change the behaviors that were degrading my health and I did. I partnered with my healthcare providers to document my improving health. This gave me confidence that the steps I was taking were producing the desired benefits. Taking the steps I took and discussed earlier has the potential to keep chronic disease at bay for most Americans. It also has the potential to save healthcare expenditures in our country that are reported to be as much as twice as high as other developed countries.

As I reported earlier, our federal government admits our system is geared toward treatment, not prevention and that 75% of current healthcare expenditures go toward **treating preventable chronic diseases** such as cardiovascular disease, type 2 diabetes and some cancers. The toll on our fellow citizens is stunning: 81 million with cardiovascular disease; 75 million with hypertension; 24 million with diabetes; 41% of the population projected to have cancer at some point; and osteoporosis afflicting 50% of women and 25% of men. We need to turn this ship in another direction.

I am not suggesting, in any way, that we turn our backs on our healthcare system. Far from it! We need our healthcare system and healthcare professionals to help us, particularly when acute problems arise and urgent medical intervention is needed. We also need proper testing and data feedback during regular check-ups. We need to understand what our test results are telling us and not wait passively for advice from our healthcare team. Do my results indicate changes need to be made? Better to make the changes before a health crisis hits.

Active engagement with your healthcare team will drive better interactions across our healthcare system. As we actively monitor our health and wellbeing **in partnership with our**

healthcare professionals, we may need to actively make lifestyle changes to enhance our health and wellness. I believe we should not be passive consumers nor should we be satisfied with a treatment mindset. Prevention is far superior but has not gotten the attention it deserves nor has it gotten the resources commensurate with its potential to help people avoid chronic diseases. We can nudge the system toward a prevention model through our regular personal interactions with our healthcare professionals.

On a personal level, we need to get more from our interactions with the healthcare system. Some preplanning will help. As I mentioned earlier, one of the most important metrics for heart health is the ratio between your triglycerides and HDL cholesterol measures. Both numbers come with a basic blood panel test. Simply divide the triglyceride number by the HDL number. This ratio is a powerful indicator and should be a regular discussion topic between you and your physician. Is it a healthy 2.0 or below? If not, what can be done to bring the number down and improve your profile? What everyday actions can be taken to lower the ratio?

When my ratio was at dangerous levels, just a few years ago, I was ignorant about the importance of this metric and my doctor did not raise the subject with me. I was in the dark and, possibly, so was my healthcare professional. This is unfortunately not uncommon, even in the Internet Age. Please understand, I am not trying to bash my doctor or the healthcare profession generally. Practicing medicine today is challenging. There are many professionals who are well informed and believe in prevention first. My basic point is — your health is way too important to hand over to anyone else. We all need to be strong advocates for ourselves and for those whose health depends on us (children and elderly relatives). Taking an active role in getting the most prevention from the system, another form of mindfulness and intention is good for us as patients and good for the system.

How can we get the most from the healthcares system? Be informed before you see your doctor. Ask questions. Write down the questions you want to discuss beforehand and get answers before you leave your doctor's office. What do the numbers on the lab test mean on a practical level? Are there other tests that need to be conducted, explained or interpreted? What am I doing right that I should continue or even increase? What lifestyle changes should I consider in light of what the medical tests are revealing?

I also recommend getting copies of full lab results and saving them in a secure place. This is critical if, as is quite common, you need to change doctors or insurance companies. Having this longitudinal data and some understanding of what it means over time will go a long way toward being a smarter healthcare consumer. Understanding your numbers over time will help identify potential chronic problems early on before they fully manifest in disease and provide you with an opportunity to pursue prevention strategies when they have the greatest benefit.

What about prescription drugs? If your healthcare professional is recommending drug therapy, especially for what appears to be a chronic condition, you need to be extra inquisitive. What are the pros and cons of the recommended drug therapy? Are there risks to consider and how significant are they? How much will the pharmaceuticals cost per day and over the course of treatment? Is there a more "conservative" course to take before embarking on drug therapy? What non-pharmaceutical alternatives are available, if any? Can the problem be addressed by lifestyle changes?

I am advocating that we take more control over our health and healthcare and insist (politely) on active partnerships with our healthcare professionals. Most healthcare professionals understand and support this model today, but if yours don't, I would find professionals who do. This will inject some healthy change into our healthcare system. If more of us follow a partnership and prevention model, healthcare professionals will respond and improve their services. We may even save some healthcare resources in the process. We would all benefit from generating healthy partnership feedback loops more broadly throughout our healthcare system.

Chapter Seventeen- The spiritual element — a way to bring more balance into our lives.

A recent PBS documentary stated that 95% people on earth believe there is a higher power behind the universe. This fundamental human belief is expressed in an astonishingly beautiful variety of ways around the globe. Organized religious communities provide a rich tapestry of belief systems and practices. They exist alongside more private manifestations of conviction that are just as satisfying to many. Some observers of this worldwide phenomena have even made the quip that "if God did not exist we would have to invent him." There appears to be a nearly universal thirst to understand life's ultimate meaning and spiritual beliefs often provide a glimpse at some helpful insights.

In one of my favorite movies, *The Big Lebowski*, the main character ("The Dude" played brilliantly by Jeff Bridges) remarked after being "introduced" to a nihilist who was passed-out in a floating pool chair with an empty bottle of bourbon nearby "... ah, that must be exhausting." According to The Dude, believing in nothing is apparently very hard work. I find it much easier and more satisfying to believe in something, especially something that provides a greater purpose to our time on earth.

My belief system is strongly informed by the observation that our world in its exquisite complexity is also well ordered. Planets move in predictable orbits according to understandable laws. Life in all its richness follows some well-established biological patterns.

The most popular and generally accepted way to explain the origin of the universe is the "Big Bang theory." According to this theory one minute there was nothing and then — Boom — everything else followed. One eminent scientist joked, "Just give us one big miracle, and we can explain all the rest." It is becoming increasingly clear to scientists that the Big Bang was a thoroughly designed event of almost impossible precision that continues to play out today as our universe expands. This idea directly challenges the view that our world derived from a series of chance events. I don't share that belief.

For example, how do we explain the exquisite genius of the human body (and other living organisms) about which we learn more every day? An honest look at any of the key attributes of our bodies surely leads to a sense of wonder. Consider our self-conscious brains; our cardiovascular system; our hearing; our sight; our ability to speak; our complex digestive system; our hormonal systems; our reproductive systems; even the elegance and complexity of a single human cell. According to scientists who study such things, the complex sequencing of the DNA that exists in every cell in our bodies (and in every living thing) defies the rules of chance to a scientific and mathematical certainty. Each of these examples (and there are many more) could rightly be considered miraculous and would justify a lifetime of study. To me, it is beyond doubt that our world is not the result of a series of random events that just happened to work out in such an extraordinary way.

One of the main ideas of this book is that evolution is a driving force in our lives and must be seriously considered in how we nourish our bodies, how we move and exercise and how we rest and recover. If any of these elements is seriously out of whack our balance is thrown off and our wellness will be degraded.

Unfortunately, evolution has become a political football. One more point for people to draw lines in the sand and hurl rhetorical bombs back and forth. This caricature of an argument is based on the false dichotomy that either evolution explains everything, including the origin of life, or is false and explains nothing. Both poles of this argument are wrong. There is another way to see evolution's key role in human life not just in the past but today.

I believe evolution is as real as gravity and shapes all life on earth. All life. But evolution does not explain how life began. In my view, the Creator of our universe set in place all natural processes from the beginning, including evolution. This is called "intelligent design" theory. The scientific evidence supporting the "design" theory and discounting the "chance" theory is compelling to me and continues to grow. My interest is not in refighting this battle. Many others have done this. The debate will continue long after we are all gone. I want to make plain my beliefs and describe how they inform and enrich my approach to life. Evolution is part of the fabric of our lives and understanding its impact on how we need to protect our health is critical.

Over the span of human history we have gained a better understanding of many natural processes, but we have much more to learn. The more we learn the more fascinating the story becomes. One of the most explosive areas of learning, and the topic of this book, is our learning about what we need to do to stay healthy.

My spiritual beliefs help me understand our world and my role in it better. They provide me a hopeful and comforting explanation of why we are here. My beliefs also provide a rationale for living life in harmonious community with others, even when no one is watching — what the ancient philosophers called virtue. For these practical reasons alone, I'm grateful to be a believer, but there are other benefits. We intuitively understand that a strong and ethical spiritual belief system supports better health and there is scientific evidence to support this view.

In *The Daniel Plan* by Pastor Rick Warren, Daniel Amen, MD and Mark Hyman, MD (with Dr. Mehmet Oz consulting) (2013) the authors present a community oriented nutrition and wellness plan based on Biblical principles. The name Daniel refers to the Old Testament story of Daniel's captivity in Babylon where he foreswore the King's food, at some personal peril, and ate only vegetables and water for ten days to demonstrate the superior healthfulness of a plant-based diet. Daniel demonstrated to one of the King's advisors that he could maintain his health and appearance better following this non-traditional path compared to his contemporaries who ate the king's normal rations. Daniel's demonstration showed that a diet of vegetables and water was superior to the finest foods available at the time to members of the king's household.

The Daniel Plan explicitly embraces a Christian-based spiritual path toward weight loss and better health. But this approach is accessible to anyone of any faith. Chapter Four is about the power of faith to support positive change in our lives. The authors believe it helps to put the ultimate power of the universe to work for you. *The Daniel Plan* also stresses that having a support system of friends and family around us leads to better results. Participants who were in groups lost twice as much weight as those who went at it alone. This is consistent with the "Roseto Effect" discussed earlier.

The Daniel Plan is rich with Biblical references to help people on their journey back to health. If these references resonate with you, put their power to work in your life. If not, feel free to overlook them. The Biblical references are not essential to the core principles of this health and nutrition lifestyle-changing plan.

At its core The Daniel Plan is very consistent in its nutrition advice with the other authors discussed in this book (with some variation at the margins). *The Daniel Plan's* advice is "Eat real, whole food. Eat a colorful variety of real, whole foods from real ingredients that you can make yourself — or that are made by another human nearby." *The Daniel Plan* at page 74. The authors go on: "Simple, real, fresh, delicious, nutrient-packed foods that are easy to cook, foods that come from a farmer's field rather than a factory, food that traveled the shortest distance from the field to your fork — that is what you should eat." *The Daniel Plan* at page 75. What should we scrupulously avoid? You guessed it: sugar, white flour, white rice and white pasta. *Id.* at pages 108-9.

Obviously, a Christian approach or even a spiritually based approach is not for everyone. Some may even find it off-putting and for that I ask your forbearance. My intent is not to convert anyone to a set of beliefs but to provide a window into one scientifically based, explicitly spiritual perspective on how to get healthier in our modern world.

Putting spiritual power to work completes my personal "toolkit" for healthy change that has been the focus of this part of the book. Next we will venture beyond these personal actions that lead to better health. I will suggest some steps we can take together to reshape the real food pyramid in America and begin to move it in a healthier direction. Changing the food landscape in our country is an effort that is urgently needed if we are to have any hope of reversing the current unhealthy trends in food consumption and the resulting growth in chronic diseases; as well as the unsustainable growth in healthcare expenditures related to treating these largely preventable conditions.

Part Four- Let's begin to reshape the real American food pyramid, improve federal nutrition policy, promote healthcare system accountability and improve formal wellness programs.

Chapter Eighteen- A review of the key population-based health trends we need to fix in the United States and increasingly throughout the developed world.

I quoted these passages earlier in Chapter Two but they are so shocking they need to be revisited.

> "The most recent data indicate that 72 percent of men and 64 percent of women are overweight or obese, with about one-third of adults being obese. Even in the absence of overweight, poor diet and physical inactivity are associated with major causes of morbidity and mortality. These include cardiovascular disease, hypertension, type 2 diabetes, osteoporosis, and some types of cancer." *Dietary Guidelines for Americans 2010* pgs. 9-10.

The American statistics are stunning: 81 million with cardiovascular disease; 75 million with hypertension; 24 million with diabetes; 41% of the population projected to have cancer at some point; and osteoporosis afflicting 50% of women and 25% of men. Clearly we are on the wrong path and need to make some changes to achieve better health for American adults. And we can't forget that there is also a growing obesity problem with America's children as detailed in Dr. Lustig's work discussed in Chapter Three. This trend will cascade into the adult numbers quoted above over time and create an even bigger problem for our country if it is not reversed.

> "As a nation [the United States], more than 75% of our health care spending is on people with chronic

conditions. These persistent conditions—the nation's leading causes of death and disability—leave in their wake deaths that could have been prevented, lifelong disability, compromised quality of life, and burgeoning health care costs." *The Power of Prevention, Chronic disease ... the public health Challenge of the 21st Century-* a report by the Center for Disease Control and Prevention (CDC), US Department of Health and Human Services (DHHS) (2009).

We have difficulty grasping the impact of health statistics that involve numbers so large that they touch almost everyone in our country. The numbers are in the multi-millions for heart disease, hypertension, diabetes, cancer and osteoporosis. Are these just statistics? No, this is a massive tragedy hiding in plain sight. These numbers almost certainly mean that every family in our country is negatively impacted at some point, often tragically. We have been lulled into thinking that these chronic diseases must be accepted along with the benefits of civilization. We have come to believe, in effect, that these diseases are inevitable. A major thesis of this book is that they are not.

We need to take a new look at the causes of these diseases and try to understand what we can do individually and together to reverse current trends. Make no mistake, these diseases — cardiovascular disease, hypertension, type 2 diabetes, osteoporosis, and some types of cancer — are not benign conditions that can be easily managed. They are killers.

I was shocked to learn recently that an older brother of a childhood friend had to have both of his feet amputated due to the debilitating effects of diabetes. I mistakenly thought this gruesome outcome was a thing of the past. I recently learned that two beloved Americans from the past also succumbed to this condition. Both the incomparable singer, Ella Fitzgerald, and the iconic baseball player, Jackie Robinson, died from diabetes. Another prominent victim of chronic disease was President Dwight "Ike" Eisenhower who died of heart disease at a fairly young age even after surviving a greatly publicized heart attack while president. This happened even though he received the best medical care available at the time of his heart attack and for the remainder of his life.

Another quote to revisit from Chapter Two... "our [American] health care system is not designed to prevent chronic illnesses." *Id.* That stark acknowledgment from our federal government should prompt some soul searching across the board. If our superbly complex, expensive and technologically advanced healthcare system is not designed for prevention, what is it designed to do? We know the answer — treatment. Treatment is a worthy endeavor. As I said in my personal story in Chapter One, modern medicine saved my life and for that I am ever grateful. But our system is tilted so far in favor of treatment that prevention does not receive the attention and resources it deserves. The costs of this model are extraordinary.

Researchers estimate that the 2014 cost of treating preventable chronic diseases in the United States will exceed $2 trillion. The amount is literally incomprehensible. This number represents almost **one out of every eight dollars** spent in our **entire economy** in a given year. And this staggering amount of healthcare spending is not making us healthier; it is generally only treating the consequences of illness. Massive spending is devoted to treating the symptoms of chronic disease, much of it preventable by our government's own accounting. Very little is being spent on preventing the most common chronic conditions before they manifest themselves.

These numbers should provoke a strong reaction but as a society we have become desensitized to the situation. Even someone with my background who worked in healthcare for 25 years and had intimate knowledge of our healthcare delivery system largely overlooked a prevention model for many years. I bought into the worldview that the healthcare system was there to address problems after they appeared. This mindset also included the belief, at some level, that as we age the chronic "diseases of civilization" were inevitable. We also receive subtle queues from various media that medical science is close to making breakthroughs that will solve any problem that currently eludes treatment. The message seems to be: we don't have to do anything different today, just hope that a cure will be available when we need it.

I have become more and more convinced that we need to strengthen our prevention efforts. Treatment is absolutely necessary but prevention is far superior. This will require a multi-pronged effort over many years. Much more needs to be done by our healthcare system in close partnership with average Americans to prevent chronic disease before it develops. And we need to do our part individually. We now have some solid scientific information about what works and what doesn't to promote wellness. It's time to put that knowledge to work individually and much more generally throughout our healthcare system. As to accepting an inevitable slow decline as we age... why should we if there is a viable alternative?

I hope the earlier Chapters have convinced you there is a better way to protect your health. At least, I hope you now understand that there may be a better approach that is worth a try. This involves personal choice and effort but we also need to enlist the help of our government and our healthcare system to put the wind at our backs. These topics will be explored more fully in the chapters ahead.

Chapter Nineteen- Putting consumer purchasing power to work to build a better American food pyramid.

I discussed the real American food pyramid earlier in Chapter Eight. The picture is not pretty. What can we do to change the situation? **We need to put our purchasing power to work.** The food industry will feel this change, discern new purchasing patterns and adapt to changing consumer behavior. This is already occurring but we can widen and accelerate the process. By supporting healthier choices with our pocket books every day, we can change the real American food pyramid over time.

This is entirely within our control whenever we shop for food or dine out. No need to get anyone else to do anything, we can do it for ourselves. Every time you shop for groceries or buy food at a restaurant, be intentional about the choices you are making. Direct your hard earned dollars toward healthier options. The food industry will take notice and make changes eventually.

The good news is that real whole food is more available than ever today. Organic produce is making inroads in regular grocery stores around the country giving us more choices than ever. Whether organic is worth the extra cost is an unfolding debate and there are different viewpoints to consider as discussed earlier. But there is little doubt that organic products are here to stay. Also, certain stores are devoting resources to consumer education about humane food production techniques. This effort is having an impact on food producers as more humane techniques are being adopted. The nationwide success of the grocery store chain Whole Foods Market® is proof of changing purchasing patterns among a growing segment of society. Our purchasing habits will help promote this change to a broader population if we spend our dollars wisely on real whole foods and deemphasize processed products. The food industry will take notice and adapt.

We can do more to accelerate these healthy trends by putting our purchasing power behind healthier choices all the time.

You can count on the data crunchers who work at the grocery store chains and large restaurant companies to collect and feed this information back to their purchasing agents. This information will in-turn travel back up the supply chain to food producers and processors. Food producers and processors will adapt their products to suit the changing consumer behavior and we all benefit from healthier nutrition over the long haul. Ultimately, through this virtuous feedback loop, the toll of chronic disease can be eased and healthcare resources preserved as we build and consume a healthier real food pyramid. Let your dollars work for your better health and together we can build a healthier future for all of us.

Chapter Twenty- Influencing government nutrition policy from the grassroots.

In my professional career, I saw from close perspective how government agencies develop and implement policy. The process is complicated and messy, to be sure, but there is a certain pattern that tends to repeat itself over and over. The pattern generally looks like this.

First, a health or nutrition "issue" (as they are labeled in government) comes into focus as a result of an unforeseen event or series of events. Or the government itself may be advocating a change to current health or nutrition policy for its own purposes or on behalf of other interested parties. A third source of these issues can be the multitude of "stakeholders" operating on the periphery of the government — think tanks, universities, healthcare systems, trade associations, media outlets, lobbyists and law firms, political parties and unions, to name a few. The stakeholders may operate in coalitions or separately. Alliances will shift depending on the issue.

The first phase — issue identification — is followed by growing urgency for the government to "do something" to solve the problem. Media and stakeholder pressure create urgency. The more intense the media and stakeholder pressure, the greater the urgency for government action. We should understand that the various media are not necessarily objective bystanders reporting on events. What the media reports, does not report and whom they rely on as experts is a robust and hotly contested field populated by savvy public relations firms and other actors influencing what makes it into print. If the precipitating event or events continues to create urgency, the interested stakeholders will use this urgency to generate pressure for government action.

Next comes the search for a plausible and politically acceptable solution. This is where the rubber meets the road. Many issues will not generate a critical mass of pressure behind a particular solution. When this happens, the issue usually fades from view. More often than not, the diverse stakeholders will have radically different viewpoints on the need for action and the preferred solution. In these situations, the opposing pressures tend to cancel each other out before a solution is implemented. At other times a high profile political battle may unfold with resolution through political decision-making at the highest levels of government. Of course, most issues are either addressed well below the public's notice or will fade away without resolution and without public attention.

So what role do average citizens have in the process I sketched out above? The reality is our ability to affect public policy as individuals is limited but not irrelevant. The different stakeholders described above are working full-time on their to-do lists of concerns. They are well funded and located at or near the seat of power in Washington, DC and the state capitols. They are professionals pursuing careers and they fight hard for the causes they support. And they are well compensated for their successes. Does that mean average citizens have no voice? No. But it suggests we need to be prudent in using our resources to influence the government on those issues we feel are important enough (the passion factor) to invest some of our precious time and effort.

One way citizens can have direct input into federal government policy is by commenting on proposed federal regulations or other initiatives. Most of us are at least somewhat aware of the difference between legislation passed by Congress and signed into law by the President that become federal statutes and the regulations written by federal agencies. They both have the force of law when final but the process of becoming law is significantly different.

When an agency seeks to write or change the law in the form of new or revised regulations it must follow the process prescribed by the federal law known as the Administrative Procedures Act. This law provides the step-by-step process agencies like the Food and Drug Administration or Agricultural Department or Health and Human Services must follow to create or change federal regulations. A key part of this process where regular citizens can have impact is when new proposed regulations (or proposed changes) are published for public comment. This publication process is carried out in the Federal Register (FR). The FR is published everyday the government is working and it is essentially a diary of the actions the federal government is taking or proposes to take.

The process I described briefly above goes on constantly. In fact, as I am writing this in February 2015 the federal government has placed a massive document before the public under the "notice and comment" requirements of the law. The government just published its *Advisory Report of the 2015 Dietary Guidelines Advisory Committee* (Committee or DGAC) in the Federal Register. This report is the step before the government proposes the new 2015 *Dietary Guidelines* (last published in 2010 and discussed earlier in this book). The request for comments states in part:

> "Written comments on the Advisory Report are encouraged from the public and will be accepted through April 8, 2015. Written public comments can be submitted and/or viewed at www.DietaryGuidelines.gov using the "Submit Comments" and "Read Comments" links, respectively. HHS and USDA requests that commenters provide a brief (250 words or less) summary of the points or issues in the comment text box. If commenters are providing literature or other resources, complete citations or abstracts and electronic links to full articles or reports are preferred instead of attaching these documents to the comment. All comments must be received by midnight (E.S.T.) on April 8, 2015, after which the time period for submitting written comments to the federal government expires. The ability to view public comments will continue to be available. Please allow until April 22, 2015, for comment submissions to be processed and posted for viewing."

In the executive summary the report states:

"The overall body of evidence examined by the 2015 DGAC identifies that a healthy dietary pattern is higher in vegetables, fruits, whole grains, low- or non-fat dairy, seafood, legumes, and nuts; moderate in alcohol (among adults); lower in red and processed meat; and low in sugar-sweetened foods and drinks and refined grains. Vegetables and fruit are the only characteristics of the diet that were consistently identified in every conclusion statement across the health outcomes. Whole grains were identified slightly less consistently compared to vegetables and fruits, but were identified in every conclusion with moderate to strong evidence. For studies with limited evidence, grains were not as consistently defined and/or they were not identified as a key characteristic. Low- or non-fat dairy, seafood, legumes, nuts, and alcohol were identified as beneficial characteristics of the diet for some, but not all, outcomes. For conclusions with moderate to strong evidence, higher intake of red and processed meats was identified as detrimental compared to lower intake. Higher consumption of sugar-sweetened foods and beverages as well as refined grains was identified as detrimental in almost all conclusion statements with moderate to strong evidence."

Note: While this report seems to be moving in the right direction, it still contains recommendations concerning whole grains (which most Americans assume they are eating when they buy products with this label but the truth is more complex). And the reality is Americans eat most grains in highly processed products that have little nutritional value and are generally known to be unhealthy as described in earlier chapters. Similarly, many believe that placing a heavy reliance on low cost legumes, which some cuisines clearly do, can also bring health problems to many people.

This request for public comments is preliminary to issuing proposed new *Guidelines* sometime in 2015. It's that simple and worth your time if you have passion around these issues.

Log on and comment away! You will have the same opportunity when the proposed *2015 Guidelines* come out.

Now, with the Internet at our fingertips, we are all placed at the virtual "seat of power" as if we were located on K Street in Washington, DC — the preferred office address of federal lobbyists. Comments received by the government must be addressed by the agency before a proposal becomes final. I have had the privilege of writing many comment letters in my career. Some achieved the results we were seeking.

Comments from regular people beyond the usual interested parties can have impact. The agencies know in advance the positions most professional commentators will take based on the institutional interests they represent and their past submissions. It is unusual for private citizens to take the time and effort to make their views known through this "notice and comment" process. Therefore, my view is that we can have real influence at this critical point in the process. The trick is finding out when the notice and comment periods are open for input on a topic you care about and making your voice heard on issues that matter to you. That is easier today than ever.

When I first started reviewing proposed regulations in the Federal Register (FR) in the early nineteen nineties I had to laboriously search a hard copy version of the FR published weekly by the government to see what issues were being raised. Our team would then have to decide whether the proposal was of sufficient importance to our organization to submit comments. Not any more. With the Internet and Google® at hand it is easy to search the FDA and USDA and HHS websites to see what regulatory proposals are pending and still open for public comment. For example following the path "FDA home> Regulatory Information> Dockets Management> Find and Comment on FDA Dockets" brings you to a page that allows a quick review of proposals and provides access to a form for commenting online. Checking these sources from time to time will keep you current and you can weigh in with your views. As I said above, it is unusual for average citizens to use this process to speak to the federal government so your comments can have impact.

Other avenues include aligning yourself with existing organizations such as the Healthy Nation Coalition. This group has taken an interest in the government's nutrition guidelines I discussed earlier. The guidelines will be revised in 2015 and comments can be sent to the drafters using the Coalition's website. This is another easy way to make your views known. It is important to make sure organizations you align with are legitimate and hold views you support. As we all know, the Internet and social media can have drawbacks. A good rule of thumb is — would I want my employer (or my Mother) to know I have supported this cause in association with this group?

Because non-affiliated citizen comment is rare, I believe such comments will garner attention and can be effective in shaping federal nutrition policy. At the very least, you will have made your voice part of the conversation — a worthwhile result in itself.

Important topics that could use our attention and input, in my opinion, are the following:

a. Government nutrition research funding — the need for more transparency and broader scope.
b. Food safety.
c. Food advertising and marketing.
d. Food labeling.
e. Food additive safety.
f. Genetically modified food safety.
g. Updating the federal nutrition guidelines, MyPyramid and MyPlate in light of current research.

If you have the energy and the passion, give it a go! You just might change the way government operates in a meaningful way.

Chapter Twenty One- It is past time to rethink some unhealthy government subsidies ($$$) provided to the food industry.

Earlier in Chapter Four, we examined some of the unhealthy food consumption trends in the United States and traced the role federal subsidies play in creating and sustaining some of these trends.

There may have been some good policy reasons behind sugar cane subsidies and corn subsidies (used to produce the sweetener HFCS) when they were instituted decades ago but we now have copious evidence proving these subsidies are making us fatter and sicker on a grand scale. Many nutrition experts believe that the massive increase in sugar consumption since the nineteen seventies is **the leading health problem** in our country. And yet this consumption is supported by dollars from the federal government under the misguided rationale that consumers should not be expected to pay the real cost of the product. This is irrationality carried to a ridiculous extreme. Unfortunately, there are strong political pressures to maintain these expenditures and without strong citizen pushback they will likely continue.

It is my view is that it is long past time to take a hard look at this spending for budgetary reasons alone. Added to the budgetary concerns is the massive negative impact on our health. This is no longer a theoretical argument. Excessive sugar consumption is a major cause of obesity and the chronic diseases of civilization that follow from being overweight. These chronic diseases add massive spending to the healthcare line items in federal and state budgets. As discussed earlier, the United States is projected to spend over $2 trillion in treating preventable chronic diseases in 2014. Government sponsored healthcare programs do much of that spending — Medicare, Medicaid, TriCare (for military retirees), VA and Indian Health Services make up the bulk of government healthcare spending (and healthcare expenditures overall) and a large proportion of those expenditures go toward treating preventable chronic diseases. The federal nutrition guidelines promulgated by the USDA and HHS appropriately recommend reducing sugar consumption. But at the same time the USDA encourages sugar and HFCS production and consumption through monetary subsidies. It really doesn't make much sense. What can we do?

Again, for those of an activist bent, I recommend that we make our voices heard in this debate. Action in the political realm is difficult and frustrating to be sure. There are many crosscurrents at work that tend to maintain the status quo. Because strong financial interests will fight any change to current spending, average citizens have a big challenge to overcome. But if we don't speak out nothing will change.

These monetary subsidies are a legislative issue controlled by the Congress. That is our first point of entry into this debate. We need to open up the lines of communication with our local Representatives. Especially those who may be involved in the House Ways and Means Committee as it has primary authority over spending bills. Communicating with Congress is easier than it has ever been. Many Congressmen and women hold regular town hall meetings. So do Senators. Their local staffs are paid to listen to your concerns and to pass them on to their bosses. Give it a go!

Find out who your representative is in the House of Representatives and Your Senators and make your voice heard. Attend a town hall meeting and speak out. It could help move this mountain.

Chapter Twenty Two- How to get more prevention from our healthcare dollars.

In earlier chapters I recommended that we become smarter consumers of healthcare. I recommended that we develop a collaborative relationship with our own healthcare providers that is focused on prevention. We have the most to lose if the healthcare system continues to pour most of its resources into treatment and the most to gain from a stronger prevention model.

Generally speaking, our healthcare payment system seeks to define "procedures" and pay a set amount each time the procedure is performed. Medicare has an intricate list of procedures that the government will pay for. The billing system demands listing of these specific procedure codes before payment is made. This model is called reimbursement.

Most private insurance plans use the Medicare fee schedule as a basis for their private contracted rates for services provided (reimbursement). Even the Medicare managed care plans (Medicare Advantage plans) have a hybrid system of monthly pre-payments that must be supported by submission of diagnoses codes each year to adjust payment amounts depending on he health status of the individual. The sicker members in the plan are, the higher the monthly payments. Therefore, both the traditional fee-for-service Medicare model (upon which most private insurance plans are based) and the Medicare managed care model tilt toward treatment or disease identification as a way to optimize provider revenue. I mention these points solely to illustrate how this system drives healthcare provider behavior toward a treatment model and away from a prevention model, not to make anyone an expert on healthcare finance.

The net result of our healthcare payment system is that providers are properly fixated on doing procedures and documenting disease diagnoses that qualify for payment. And since providers are rational economic actors they tend to gravitate toward activities that will optimize their revenue within the bounds of the law.

What can we do as healthcare consumers to shift the focus to prevention and away from treatment?

Health insurance companies, government health care programs and employers pay the bills for healthcare in America. Actually, we all pay the bills indirectly but these agents pay on our behalf. When is the last time you let your insurance company know your thoughts on anything other than paying bills? If a government program covers you, do you know what the program is doing to promote prevention? Does your employer health plan really promote employee health? Is the commitment to employee health supported by significant resources or is it a check-the-box type commitment?

Again, we need to be more active in urging our health insurance companies, government health care programs and employers to do more to keep us healthy before chronic disease comes calling. Some of the personal steps recommended earlier come in to the mix. On a practical level, what kind of food is in the break room at work— donuts, pizza or candy? Does your daily work schedule allow for increased movement or exercise breaks? Does your health insurance company or government health care program have an active program for wellness promotion? This topic is next.

Chapter Twenty Three- Building better wellness programs.

Most of us receive our healthcare coverage from either employer-based health plans or government sponsored plans. Both of these institutions rely on health insurance companies to document coverage policies, organize healthcare delivery networks and pay the bills. The large insurance companies that underwrite this coverage have gone through major consolidations over the last twenty years. In plain language, that means there are now a handful of very large national companies and a few strong regional players. These large companies tend to provide remarkably similar products and services based on established programs that make economic sense to them and that are acceptable to regulators at both the state and federal levels. The regulators have enormous power to dictate how these companies do business even down to establishing limits on profit margins and specific benefit requirements. The Affordable Care Act of 2010 increased this regulatory involvement. The effects of this new law are becoming clearer to consumers as time passes and it will be interesting to see how this law evolves.

Health insurance products must meet established regulatory criteria and must be pre-approved before they are offered to the public. This makes sense because consumers are not in a position to evaluate complex coverage issues and the appropriate cost of health insurance products. However, this oversight is expensive and cumbersome and even arbitrary at times. This leads to a sluggish situation where products and services change very slowly, if at all.

Innovation in this environment is challenging but not impossible. My view is we need to get much more support from the healthcare insurance companies and government programs and employers geared toward real wellness.

As I have previously discussed the American healthcare system devotes three quarters of every dollar to **treating** preventable chronic diseases. I have argued earlier that we need to seek out and partner with healthcare providers who emphasize prevention over treatment. Wellness programs are an important component of prevention but there is even more that these programs can achieve.

I would argue that "wellness" is a higher standard of performance for our healthcare system than prevention. Prevention is absolutely critical but, as consumers, we should not stop there. We need to agitate (again politely) for more robust "wellness" programs. Wellness is a term of art in the health insurance industry that has come to encompass smoking cessation, weight loss, basic nutrition and similar programs. Usually there is a dash of nutrition and exercise advice thrown in along the way. Some insurance programs provide discounted gym memberships as a wellness benefit. These programs are a good start but are they having the desired impact?

My experience tells me our personal journeys toward wellness could use greater support from the insurance companies (and government programs) that manage healthcare spending in our country. I would ask each of us to answer a few simple questions:

- Does your healthcare insurance company have a wellness program?
- Do you participate in this program in a meaningful way?
- Has the program helped you get healthier?
- What medical data supports your conclusion that you are healthier as a result of your wellness program?
- Does your insurance company publicize results of their formal wellness programs?
- Are the results based on process measures (how many classes attended, how many enrollees, how many tests completed, etc.) or health outcomes (documented health improvements)?

This last question may seem technical but is the most important one we need to understand. Many "quality measures" that have been developed over the past thirty years are process oriented. How many flu shots given per 100 enrollees? How many smoking cessation programs provided per 100 enrollee smokers? How many weight loss classes presented per 100 enrollees? And so on. These process measurements are important but they don't measure the impact, i.e. the health improvement outcome, of the process being measured.

Health outcomes measures get more to the heart of the matter. We now have the technology to measure health outcomes that matter and compare data from large populations against other comparable large populations and draw meaningful conclusions. The outcomes that matter most are the incidence and mortality attributable to the chronic diseases that have been the focus of this book: obesity, hypertension, type 2 diabetes, cardiovascular disease, heart attack and certain cancers. A truly robust "wellness" program should be able to document improvement of these critical health outcomes and link it back to the wellness program.

How can we help build formal wellness programs that work? It is my view that the insurance companies will not move much beyond the status quo unless we, as consumers, demand more. And we need to hold our insurers to measurable outcomes improvement. This suggests greater consumer involvement to create increased demand on the healthcare system for real world solutions that measurably help people attain better health and wellness outcomes, not just process measures (as important as some of them are).

I have explored a scientifically based nutrition and exercise approach in this book that works for me; and that has worked for many people. The basics of this approach are not new. Still, many healthcare providers and many health insurance companies are unaware of the benefits of this approach and continue to recommend approaches that have not worked for our society as a whole. The bureaucratic inertia around the outmoded advice to "eat better and exercise more" has been remarkably resistant to new evidence. We can help change this pattern by demanding more from our healthcare insurance providers.

Many larger employers provide "wellness" programs through the office. These programs are to be applauded but should also be evaluated using outcomes criteria suggested above. Is the program helping people increase or maintain their motivation to get healthier? Is the program broad-based or do only the healthier employees participate? How easy is it to participate? Is it cost effective? Is the program producing the desired health improvements?

By taking a greater interest in wellness programs that may already be available to us through our insurance providers, government programs or through work we can move the needle on our personal wellness. We can also help these programs get better by providing knowledgeable feedback on the substance of the programs and the need for robust outcome measures.

Summary and Final Thoughts- Recapture your birthright and optimize your health and wellness.

Our natural birthright is to be healthy and vital.

This birthright has been handed down to us by our ancient ancestors who faced danger almost every day and had to work hard for their daily nutrition. Overcoming these challenges using their brains and their brawn allowed them to thrive over millions of years of evolutionary development and adaptation to become our Paleolithic forebears. Life was challenging for these "Paleos" but they were resourceful and healthy. Ultimately their descendents, all of us, populated the entire globe.

Agriculture emerged as a great gift around 10,000 years ago that allowed civilization to flourish. But this gift also brought unforeseen negative consequences to our health that have grown more pressing in recent years. This book explored some of these negatives.

But this is not a story of doom and gloom. Researchers are beginning to understand some of the causes of our modern chronic health problems and we now have better strategies today to head off these chronic diseases before they strike.

The primary purpose of this book is to introduce you to research and resources that offer scientifically valid explanations for the modern scourge of the chronic "diseases of civilization" and offer scientifically sound evolution-based solutions for healthy nutrition and effective exercise.

In Chapters Five through Seventeen, we explored the best information available today to help you build your personal "toolbox" for optimal wellness. What are the tools?

- Let an evolutionary perspective guide your nutrition and exercise worldview
- Calorie counting and excessive cardio exercise do not work

- Nutrition — eat real whole food and pass on the processed stuff
- Exercise — do more intense but shorter strength and interval training
- Move more — walk, walk, walk
- Play
- Low carbohydrate diets are effective and there are a number of options available — chose one that fits you and put it to work
- Be intentional about food shopping
- Have fun preparing and enjoying food with your family and others
- Evaluate food quality and make informed cost-based purchasing decisions
- Take steps to bust through chronic stress
- Build better personal relationships at work and at home
- Get restful sleep as often as possible
- Become smarter healthcare consumers
- Tend to the spiritual side of your nature

This is putting **Evolution Health** to work for your benefit and the benefit of the people you love. These tools are totally under your control. Experience shows that motivation is the key to success. If motivation falters, trouble looms. I have offered some ideas on how to generate initial motivation and lock-in success over the long haul. I hope these ideas prove valuable to you.

In Chapters Eighteen through Twenty Three, I offered some thoughts on how we could take steps beyond personal action to obtain optimal wellness and begin to make positive changes in our country. I strongly believe we need to begin to improve those government nutrition policies that negatively impact societal health, move our vast healthcare system toward prevention and improve existing "wellness" programs offered by healthcare insurers and employers. What are the tools for this project?

- Put consumer purchasing power to work to build a better real food pyramid

- Take grassroots action to influence government nutrition policy
- Take grassroots action to reduce unhealthy government food subsidies
- Demand outcomes-based results from wellness programs offered to you by healthcare insurers, government sponsored healthcare programs and employers

These latter suggestions are offered for those people who have the passion and the energy.

We have power and can make a difference. It takes action though. I intend to do my part. I hope some of you will join me. Our country needs more informed voices to join the conversation if we are ever going to change course to overcome the epidemic of chronic diseases and move toward a healthier future.

My Personal Wellness Guidelines

These guidelines flow directly from my research and personal experience. They are the guidelines I follow in my own life.

There are many definitions of "wellness" but let's keep it simple. You know when you feel well and you know when you don't feel well. Let that guide you in what you eat and how you exercise day to day and over the long term.

These guidelines are derived and synthesized from three research sources: 1) archeological and anthropological study of the foods our healthy, pre-agricultural ancestors consumed and their daily movements, 2) study of the diets of modern day hunter-gatherers, and 3) modern medical, genetic and nutritional research. None of this research is original with me, as I have described in the book, but comes from the most persuasive information I discovered in my search for some practical steps I could take to improve my own health.

Our pre-agricultural ancestors lived and thrived during the millions of years before the agricultural revolution, when our genetic makeup was gradually being formed through evolution. Modern day hunter-gatherers (sadly a vanishing breed) are also healthy and energetic, eating what they can hunt and gather in their local areas. Mimicking their diets of locally available wild meats, wild fish, vegetables, fruits, nuts and seeds; and avoiding sugar and processed foods has the potential to return us to optimal health at any age. We also have the advantage of modern medical, genetic and nutritional research to guide us in our search for healthy foods that fit our genetic makeup. If we add some sensible regular exercise and more movement to our daily routines, we are on the way to recovering our birthright — real wellness.

THE FOLLOWING NUTRITION GUIDELINES CAN BE SUMMARIZED IN ONE SENTENCE: EAT REAL, WHOLE FOOD AND SKIP THE PROCESSED STUFF!

Put these healthy items on your menu:

- reasonable portions (4-6 ounces) of healthy protein, including lean grass-fed meats and free range fowl, wild fish (especially wild salmon) and other proteins rich in omega-3 fatty acids,
- fresh eggs (omega-3 enriched and/or cage-free),
- unlimited non-starchy vegetables, especially the green leafy ones,
- fruit (with some restraint due to the high natural sugar content of some fruits if the main goal is weight loss),
- shellfish (clams, oysters, shrimp, mussels, lobster and abalone),
- sea vegetables (seaweed),
- nuts and seeds (with some restraint due to their high caloric content if the main goal is weight loss),
- mushrooms, especially Maitake, Shiitake and Reishi; Portobello and Cremini (more mature white button mushrooms),
- water when you are thirsty (you don't need 8 glasses a day because whole foods supply much of the water you need),
- tea and coffee without sugar added (both healthy antioxidants),
- extra virgin olive oil (EVO), coconut oil and other healthy oils for flavoring and cooking,
- herbs and spices for flavoring (unlimited),
- butter (from grass fed cows is best, but pricey),
- high quality natural cheeses from cows, sheep and goats (raw, unpasteurized, naturally aged),
- non-starchy tubers like yams and sweet potatoes, but not standard potatoes that tend to be very starchy and not as nutritious,
- quinoa (a healthy legume, pronounced "keen-wah")
- dark chocolate with at least 70% cacao as an occasional treat (not milk or white chocolate or chocolate candy bars),

- red wine- up to one or two 4 ounce glasses per day depending on body size and if you can consume alcohol responsibly,
- an occasional distilled spirit cocktail without added sugar or salt if you can consume alcohol responsibly.

The following foods are fine on occasion, but should not be over-consumed:
- wild rice and brown rice in small portions,
- legumes (beans, lentils, peas, soy products and peanuts). Legumes can mimic the unhealthy effects of cereal grains in some people. Legumes are an inferior source of protein and should not be a mainstay of your diet. Having them from time to time is fine. However, if they don't agree with you, better to leave them off your menu.

These foods should be off your menu most of the time, but do not need to be avoided completely:
- starchy tubers (especially regular "Idaho" potatoes),
- high-quality restaurant produced fried foods,
- processed dairy products (high quality dairy products are OK at any time),

You should take these commonly consumed items off your menu for good- LISTED IN PRIORITY WITH WORST FIRST:
- refined sugar and High Fructose Corn Syrup (HFCS)- one or both are in almost all processed foods and sweetened drinks such as sodas, teas, sport drinks, etc,
- trans fats- still contained in many processed foods (e.g. frozen dinners, baked goods and margarine) and used by fast food outlets to deep fry things like fried chicken, French fries and donuts,
- processed carbohydrates from cereal grains, especially modern wheat, processed into bread, rolls, pastries, pasta, donuts, tortillas (wheat or corn), chips and other snack food;
- refined white rice- turns into blood sugar faster than real sugar,

- processed foods- anything in a box or a bag with a long list of unintelligible ingredients (these are the items shelved in the interior aisles and near the check-out counters of most grocery stores),
- poor quality oils- canola, corn, cottonseed, peanut, safflower, soybean and sunflower; and generic vegetable oil,
- fast food- generally loaded with salt, sugar, processed grains and poor quality vegetable oils,
- added salt- many foods contain natural salt that can satisfy our taste for salt without overloading our systems,
- artificial sweeteners- these tend to trigger cravings for other sugary sweet things,
- pasteurized products, including cow's milk and most processed fruit juices,
- beer- a fattening beverage derived from fermented cereal grains that contains gluten. (Gluten free beer has not obtained much traction in the marketplace.)

TO HEALTHIER NUTRITON, ADD
- Reasonable regular exercise and increased daily movement.
- Activities that lift your spirits, reduce stress, and relax the mind and body, such as, laughter, massage, yoga, meditation, tai chi, nature walks and play (its not just for children and pets).
- Restful sleep with a natural wake up as often as possible.

GETTING STARTED- THE BUILDING BLOCKS

- Ask for and obtain the support of your family and/or a small group.
- Clean out the processed food from your refrigerator, pantry and work areas.
- Shop intentionally; buy real, whole food.

- Read labels on all processed products- they can be tricky, even deceptive. If you don't understand what the label is telling you, best to leave it on the shelf.
- Prepare and cook your own real, whole food. Get some basic cookbooks or information online.
- Be creative.
- Discover new foods and recapture your taste buds.
- Prepare food and cook as a family.
- Enjoy mealtime together (turn off the TV).
- Savor your food while eating.
- Be mindful.
- Have fun.

THE ESSENTIAL PILLARS OF SUCCESS (SCARF)

- SUPPORT- OBTAIN SUPPORT FROM YOUR FAMILY AND/OR A SMALL GROUP.
- COMMITMENT- FOLLOW THE GUIDELINES FOR FORTY DAYS AND ASSESS HOW YOU ARE DOING.
- ATTITUDE- ACCEPT THAT CHANGE IS DIFFICULT. DON'T SEEK PERFECTION, THAT WILL ONLY INCREASE HARMFUL STRESS.
- RESOURCES- LEARN THE GUIDELINES AND USE THEM DAILY.
- FLEXIBILITY- FOLLOW THE 80/20 RULE- STAY WITH IT AT LEAST 80% OF THE TIME. IF YOU OCCASIONALLY STRAY, ALLOW YOURSELF FORGIVENESS AND THEN GET BACK ON THE PATH TO WELLNESS.

Legal Disclaimer: **This is not medical advice.** Only a trained and licensed healthcare provider with knowledge of your health status can provide valid medical advice. This information is intended to be considered in conjunction with the medical and nutrition advice you are already receiving from qualified professionals. You are responsible for your own health and need to work with your healthcare professionals on medical questions. These guidelines are meant to provide information for you to consider in light of your life experiences and health status. **The legal responsibility, legal**

accountability and consequences of implementing these guidelines in whole or in part are yours. Work in partnership with your existing healthcare professionals on the advisability of adopting some or all of these guidelines in your daily routines.

APPENDIX B- RESOURCES

PRIMARY RESOURCES

The Primal Blueprint by Mark Sisson (2009 hard cover; updated paperback edition 2012)- by far the best Primal/Paleo book on the market, especially for those over 50 (the author recently turned 60). Clearly written with summaries at the beginning and end of each chapter. Great graphics. An innovative approach to exercise that is easy and provides effective workout suggestions involving more intense strength and interval training that can be completed in about 20 minutes per session a few times per week — no more endless cardio workouts.

The Calorie Myth by Jonathan Bailor (2014) based on a decade long review of the scientific literature of nutrition and health that refutes many common beliefs (myths) about nutrition, exercise and wellness and provides specific advice on what the best science advises us to do.

The Paleo Diet by Loren Cordain, PhD (hardcover 2002; updated paperback 2013)- this book launched the modern Paleo movement. Dr. Cordain is an academic researcher who has devoted the last 30 years to understanding the habits of our hunter-gatherer ancestors (Paleolithic peoples) and putting that wisdom down for modern use in a "just the facts" manner based on sound scientific data.

The Paleo Solution by Robb Wolf (2010)- a witty retelling of Robb's journey from being a sickly vegetarian to a healthy Paleo, with a heavy emphasis on the problems associated with grain consumption. Also provides extensive exercise advice.

Living Low Carb by Jonney Bowden, PhD, CNS (2013)- reviews the top 23 low carbohydrate diets and explains how they might work, or not work, for different personality types. This simplifies the job of choosing a diet/lifestyle plan that might work for you from among the thousands out in the commercial marketplace.

The Daniel Plan by Pastor Rick Warren, Daniel Amen, MD and Mark Hyman, MD (2013)- a community based nutrition and wellness plan based on Biblical principles.

Paleo Comfort Foods by Julie & Charles Mayfield (2011)- a visually attractive cookbook that describes all the tools you need to set up a kitchen and cook healthy food with style and variety.

Make it Paleo by Bill Staley and Hayley Mason (2011)- Easy to follow recipes even for beginner cooks. Contains many of your childhood favorites.

OTHER RESOURCES

Grain Brain by David Perlmutter, MD with Kristin Loberg (2013)- Subtiled "The surprising truth about wheat, carbs and sugar- your brain's silent killers." #1 NY Times bestseller.

Wheat Belly by William Davis, MD (2014 paperback version)- Subtitled "Lose the wheat, lose the weight, and find your path back to health." More than one million copies sold.

The 150th Healthiest Foods on Earth by Jonny Bowden, PhD (2007). Visually attractive and loaded with the reasons why these foods make his "best of" list. Generally consistent with a Paleo/Primal based nutrition philosophy.

Eat It to Beat It by David Zinczenko (2013). This New York Times bestselling author provides a clever walk through the chain restaurant's offerings and the processed food found in a typical grocery store. This book takes a contrarian view of processed foods and tries to sort out the OK from the truly awful, based on calorie count on the not unreasonable assumption that most people will eat a lot of these foods in any given week. His solution is "moderation." Personally I am skeptical that this approach will work. That said, the book is valuable because it provides practical information about the endless and very tricky ways the food industry formulates and labels its products and some really scary information about some unusual ingredients that some processed foods contain. Some of the massive calorie counts for some of the offerings are truly astounding. My view is to skip the entire category of processed food and eat real whole food so you know what you are eating and not taking someone else's word for it.

The Great Cholesterol Myth by Jonny Bowden, PhD and Steven Sinatra, MD (2012). This book debunks the belief that "high cholesterol" is a problem and demonstrates why statins are the wrong answer to the wrong question for most people.